The
CHEESE
TRAP

The
CHEESE
TRAP

How Breaking a Surprising Addiction
Will Help You Lose Weight,
Gain Energy, *and* Get Healthy

Neal D. Barnard, MD, FACC

Recipes by Dreena Burton
Foreword by Marilu Henner

GRAND CENTRAL
Life & Style

NEW YORK · BOSTON

Copyright © 2017 by Neal D. Barnard, MD
Recipes copyright © 2017 by Dreena Burton

Jacket design by Faceout Studio/Jeff Miller
Jacket photographs © Shutterstock

Cover copyright © 2017 by Hachette Book Group, Inc.

Grand Central Life & Style
Hachette Book Group
1290 Avenue of the Americas, New York, NY 10104
grandcentrallifeandstyle.com
twitter.com/grandcentralpub

First Edition: February 2017

Grand Central Life & Style is an imprint of Grand Central Publishing. The Grand Central Life & Style name and logo are trademarks of Hachette Book Group, Inc.

The publisher is not responsible for websites (or their content) that are not owned by the publisher.

The Hachette Speakers Bureau provides a wide range of authors for speaking events. To find out more, go to www.hachettespeakersbureau.com or call (866) 376-6591.

Limburger cartoon (page 11) is copyright © Jen Sorensen.

Dairy farming illustrations (pages 124, 125, and 126) are copyright © Food and Agriculture Organization of the United Nations, 2008. *Small-Scale Dairy Farming Manual*, http://www.fao.org/docrep/011/t1265e/t1265e.htm. Reproduced with permission.

Tofu "Feta" (page 217) and Coconut Bacon (page 232) recipes are copyright © Dreena Burton and are reprinted from *Plant-Powered Families* with permission by BenBella Books.

Library of Congress Cataloging-in-Publication Data has been applied for.

ISBNs: 978-1-4555-9468-9 (hardcover); 978-1-4555-9466-5 (ebook)

Printed in the United States of America

LSC-C

10 9 8 7 6 5 4 3 2 1

Contents

Foreword

I was caught in the Cheese Trap.

For years, I was the girl whose idea of a gourmet meal was a pot of cheese fondue followed by cheesecake. I would think nothing of spending three days chipping away at a pound of Jarlsberg, eating no other food, and proudly calling it my "1,700-Calories-a-Day Diet"! Every two weeks for several months at a time, I would stop at Zabar's on my way to unemployment to buy what they called "Cheese Ends," which was nothing more than what was left over after they cut up blocks of cheese. Five different little chunks in every bag, and I'd buy at least five bags with my hard-earned unemployment dollars. I was not only unemployed; I was also fat, constipated, and had pimples. My skin was puffy and toxic looking. I weighed 54 pounds more than I do today. And I was so intestinally clogged that I had to spend time in a clinic because I hadn't been able to "take out the trash" for seventeen days. Seventeen days of constipation.

All because of cheese.

Not milk. (I never had a full glass.)

Not yogurt. (Not my thing.)

Not cottage cheese. (Yuck.)

It was the cheese. And I craved it every day.

I can honestly say that the single most important step I took in my health journey was giving up dairy products—cheese, in particular. I had been voraciously reading about the effects of different foods on your body because I had lost my parents at an early age and needed a way to make sense of their deaths. I was seventeen when my father died of a heart attack at fifty-two, and I was barely twenty-six when my mother succumbed to the ravages of rheumatoid arthritis. She was fifty-eight. I knew my health needed improving, so I started making changes. But nothing had quite the impact on my health like giving up cheese. In fact, I consider the day I gave up cheese forever—Wednesday, August 15, 1979—my true health birthday. This was the day when everything I had been reading about dairy products came together, and it finally hit me: *The only thing dairy is supposed to do is turn a 50-pound calf into a 300-pound cow in six months. (If those are your aspirations, knock yourself out!) A human being has twenty-seven feet of intestines and one stomach, while a baby calf has nine feet of intestines and four stomachs! Why are we drinking cow's or goat's milk and not orangutan milk—our closest mammal relative? And you would never make cheese from the breast milk of your next-door neighbor, but you are sucking from the udder of a cow you don't even know! And cheese is even worse! More concentrated and full of salt and bacteria. What was I thinking?*

When I gave up dairy, everything about me changed.

My skin cleared, my cheeks de-puffed, my nose narrowed, my eyes brightened, my body streamlined.

Gone was the bloated feeling after eating. And the sore throats and colds I'd gotten four times a year since I was a kid. Mucus was no longer coursing through my body, clogging my sinuses, pores, and digestive tract. The "spare tire" I thought was going to be there forever disappeared, because I was finally able to take out the trash. Every. Single. Day. (And then some!) I stopped yo-yo dieting because I was no longer taxing my body by ingesting a food it wasn't designed to break down. I dropped the extra weight in a healthy way, and I've kept it off since that fateful day in 1979. Everything else improved, too, including my attitude, sleeping habits, speaking, singing, breathing, and breath. I no longer felt a general malaise. It was as if a fog lifted and I could think more clearly, all because I was no longer held prisoner by my cheese addiction. I was no longer an unsuspecting "mouse" caught in the Cheese Trap!

I've known Dr. Neal Barnard for over fifteen years as the best resource for great cutting-edge health and medical information. There is no one better at taking dry, esoteric scientific data and making it not only understandable, but also entertaining! Time and again I've seen him captivate an audience by walking them through a process from what they think they know about a subject to a greater understanding that stays with them years later. His images and explanations are so simple, yet so profound, you know you will be using them to explain to other people why you might have made a certain health choice.

In this remarkable book, you will learn everything you've ever wanted to know about cheese and why it's got such a stranglehold on most of us. Dr. Barnard has broken down all of the research and food science in such a way that you will never look at another piece of Cheddar, Swiss, or mozzarella in the same way again. All cheeses will be gone for Gouda! (Sorry, I couldn't resist!)

Dr. Barnard not only explains what's in cheese and why it's so addictive; he also walks you through the cheese-making process from the animals' and manufacturers' points of view and how it's become the industry giant it is today. As usual, Dr. Barnard leaves no stone unturned, and the world is a better place for it.

So if you want to be healthier, happier, and look like the animal you were meant to be—because you are no longer ingesting a product from the mother's milk of an animal you have nothing to do with—then this is the book for you! And if you know someone who snores, gets sore throats and colds, fights their weight, deals with hormonal imbalances, please give them a copy, too!

—Marilu Henner,
actress, *New York Times* bestselling author,
radio host, and health advocate

A Note to the Reader

I hope this book provides you with new insights on food and health and more than a few interesting facts to share. Before we begin, let me mention two important points:

See your health care provider. Health problems can be serious business. If you are making a diet change—and I hope you are—it is a good idea to talk with your doctor along the way. This is not because changing your diet is dangerous. Quite the opposite. It is a really good idea. But people who are taking medications—for diabetes or high blood pressure, for example—very often need to adjust their medications when they improve their diets. Sometimes, they are able to discontinue their drugs altogether. Do not do this on your own. Work with your health care provider to reduce or discontinue your medicines if and when the time is right.

Also, talk with your doctor before you jump into a new exercise routine. If you have been sedentary, have any serious health problems, have a great deal of weight to lose, or are over forty, have your provider check whether you are ready for exercise, and how rapidly to begin.

Get complete nutrition. The way of eating presented in this book is likely to improve your nutrition overall, in addition to the specific health benefits it may bring. Even so, you will want to ensure that you get complete nutrition. Please read the details in Chapter 9. In particular, be sure to take a daily multiple vitamin or other reliable source of vitamin B_{12}, such as fortified cereals or fortified soy milk. Vitamin B_{12} is essential for healthy nerves and healthy blood.

Acknowledgments

I am very grateful to the many people who helped make this book a reality. Dreena Burton created the wonderful recipes, and Amber Green, RD, analyzed each one for its nutrient content. Adam Drewnowski of the University of Washington; Patrick Fox of Ireland's University College Cork; Michael Tunick, PhD, from the U.S. Department of Agriculture; and Fred Nyberg, PhD, dean of the Faculty of Pharmacy, Uppsala University, Uppsala, Sweden, provided answers on key scientific issues.

Nanci Alexander, owner of Fort Lauderdale's legendary Sublime restaurant, revealed her secrets for building a completely dairy-free menu. Michael Schwarz, Miyoko Schinner, and Tal Ronnen kindly shared their wisdom on the rewards and challenges of replacing cheese, and Geno Vento shared an insider's look at the restaurant world. Many others—identified here mostly by their first names—shared their personal experiences with cheese and the benefits of making a diet change. I am especially grateful to our research participants who have put up with many late-evening meetings, needle sticks, and examinations in order to clarify how foods affect health.

At the Physicians Committee for Responsible Medicine, Dania DePas, Jessica Frost, and our communications team, along with

Rose Saltalamacchia, Cael Croft, Jill Eckart, and many other Physicians Committee staffers, have done a phenomenal job of spreading the word far and wide. Mindy Kursban and Mark Kennedy worked long and hard to keep the food industry and the government honest and accountable. Rosendo Flores was extraordinarily helpful in finding and sharing research documents. Thanks to Ashley Waddell, Reina Podell, Bonnie MacLeod, Laura Anderson, Erica Springer, and Zeeshan Ali for reviewing the manuscript.

And I owe a huge debt of gratitude to my literary agent, Brian DeFiore; my editor, Sarah Pelz; and the team at Grand Central for all they have done to make sure this book would reach the people who need to see it. Thank you!

Hidden in Plain Sight

Does this sound familiar? You'd like to lose a few pounds, but you're having trouble, and it's hard to figure out why. Your eating habits are really not too bad. Maybe you're not exercising quite as much as you'd like, but you're not entirely sedentary either. And still, it's a challenge to lose weight.

Or maybe you have a health condition that is just not getting better: high cholesterol, high blood pressure, diabetes, sore joints, headaches, or less-than-healthy-looking skin. What could be causing the problem?

The answer could be hiding in plain sight.

Imagine losing weight easily, week by week, month by month, without counting calories—and without adding one minute of exercise. Imagine your friends asking how you succeeded at trimming away all those pounds. Imagine them telling you how great you look. Imagine your cholesterol improving, your blood pressure getting better, and your health rebounding day by day.

If you're looking to revamp your eating habits to lose weight or improve your health, the place to start is not with sugar, carbs, or processed foods. The place to start is with cheese.

You love cheese. But I'm sorry to tell you, it does not love you back. And the sooner you recognize it, the sooner you'll conquer your weight or health problems.

"No way!" you might be thinking. "That's impossible!"

Think again. Cheese packs a surprising number of calories—more than enough to explain the weight that you have gained over the years. And what cheese makers did not tell you is that cheese harbors mild opiates that might be just strong enough to keep you hooked. That "fattening-addictive" combination is what makes cheese a serious problem for your weight.

And it gets worse. Because cheese comes from a cow—often a *pregnant* cow—you are getting a dose of estrogens—female sex hormones—that you never bargained for. And cheese makers add enough salt to make cheese one of the highest-sodium foods. It is high in saturated fat and cholesterol, too. Loaded with calories, high in sodium, packing more cholesterol than steak, and sprinkled with hormones—if cheese were any worse, it would be Vaseline.

"What!?" you are now asking. "Cheese? There's no way it could be that fattening. And to call it addictive is ridiculous! And besides, I love cheese."

Hold that thought.

First of all, you don't need to give up that taste—you just need healthier ways to get it, and I'll show them to you. But, yes, cheese is more fattening—by far—than bread, potatoes, or even pure sugar. Here's why: Most of the calories—about 70 percent—in typical cheeses come from fat, and every last fat gram packs 9 calories.

Compare that to sugar: It turns out that pure sugar has only

4 calories per gram. And to turn sugar into fat, your body has to completely rearrange the sugar molecules; that process burns off another quarter of its calories, or thereabouts.

That's not to say that sugar is health food. But cheese fat has more than twice the calories found in the most concentrated sugar, and its calories are easily stored on your belly, around your thighs, under your chin, and everywhere else. You can see them and feel them, and they show up on the scale.

And what about that addictive effect? Not only does cheese have the saltiness and mouthfeel that some people crave, but as cheese is digested, it releases special chemicals, called *caso-morphins.* In the brain, these chemicals attach to the same opiate receptors that heroin or morphine attach to. Don't get me wrong—casomorphins are nowhere near as mind-numbing as illegal narcotics. But, like heroin and morphine, casomorphins are indeed opiates that affect the brain.

Think of it this way: Coffee contains caffeine, a mild stimulant. While caffeine is not as powerful as, say, amphetamines, it is still strong enough to keep you hooked, as any coffee drinker will tell you. Casomorphins have subtle brain effects, too. And evidence shows that they can keep you hooked, too.

Some foods are fattening. Others are addictive. Cheese is both—fattening *and* addictive. And that's the problem.

Does it matter? It sure does. Look at the numbers: An average American eats more than 33 pounds of cheese every year. Now imagine if just one and a half of those 33 pounds showed up on the scale each year (which, in fact, happens to be the amount of weight the average American gains each year). Over a decade, that adds up to 15 unwanted pounds, and 30 pounds every two decades. Sound familiar? That's more than enough to explain the weight epidemic in the U.S.

All the Taste, None of the Regrets

A surprising number of health problems are linked to cheese and other dairy products. If your cholesterol is high, could it be because cheese is a huge source of cholesterol-boosting saturated fat, as well as cholesterol itself? If your blood pressure is up, could it be because cheese is also loaded with blood pressure–raising sodium, plus enough fat that it makes your heart push harder to pump your blood? If you have diabetes, could it be that the "bad fat"—saturated fat—that predominates in cheese is causing the insulin resistance that is the hallmark of this condition?

If you have rheumatoid arthritis or any other autoimmune condition, could it be that dairy proteins—which are highly concentrated in cheese—are triggering your symptoms? And what about the hormone effects of cheese? In this book, we will cover all of these and much more.

Filled with fat, crammed with cholesterol, and steeped in sodium, cheese is a seriously unhealthy product. Its addictive properties keep you hooked, even while it works its mischief on your waistline and damages your health.

But here's the good news. I will show you how to slim down and dramatically improve your health by gaining control over this gooey yellow monster. Yes, there are ways to get the taste of cheese, with none of the regrets.

I'll show you how to make the best lasagna, the most delicious pizza, a perfect sandwich topping, a mac and cheese that will delight any twelve-year-old, and many, many other wonderfully tasty foods. You'll know exactly which foods to choose when you're dining out, whether you are at a Michelin-starred restaurant or a fast-food spot. As you savor these delicious foods, you'll almost feel your waistline trimming, your cholesterol and blood pressure coming down, and your health improving.

Most importantly, you will look at foods very differently. Some give you a health boost, while others get in your way, and now you'll know exactly which are which, and you'll take that power into your day-to-day life.

Real People, Real Results

In this book, you will meet people whose lives have been transformed. Patricia suffered with stubborn weight problems, diabetes, and worsening heart disease until she discovered that a simple diet change could trim away 95 pounds and make her feel great. Marc had a similar experience. His extra weight melted away, as did diabetes, hypertension, cholesterol problems, and erectile dysfunction. He got his life back.

Katherine, an aerospace engineer, was at the point of needing a hysterectomy to treat endometriosis, a hormone-related condition that causes intractable abdominal pain and can threaten fertility. Breaking a love affair with cheese and other unhealthful foods cured her pain, trimmed her waistline, and let her live again.

Lauren, an attorney, suffered with crushing migraines. Once she discovered that her headaches were triggered by dairy proteins, she had more power than a prescription could deliver. Migraines? Gone!

Ann suffered from respiratory problems and a chronically out-of-sorts digestive tract. She was the daughter of a milk processor, so dairy products were the last thing she imagined would have been the cause of her problems. But when a doctor suggested going dairy-free, her problems disappeared.

You will also meet some people in the cheese industry who have devoted countless hours and millions of dollars to keeping you hooked on cheese—people who have signed surprising financial arrangements with restaurant chains to, in so many words, *trigger cheese cravings*. And you will meet innovators, like Michael Schwarz, Miyoko Schinner, and Tal Ronnen, who have devised delightful savory cheeses from healthful, entirely plant-based ingredients, with none of the moo or goo of dairy cheeses. You'll meet restaurateurs like Nanci Alexander, whose gourmet restaurant replaced *all* the cheese with truly exquisite ingredients that keep customers coming back for more. They are revolutionizing the world of food.

Let me also introduce myself. I grew up in Fargo, North Dakota, and went to medical school at the George Washington University in Washington, DC, and am on the faculty there today. In 1985, I founded the Physicians Committee for Responsible Medicine to bring a new emphasis on prevention and nutrition into medical practice and to improve how research is conducted.

Over the years, the Physicians Committee has completed many research studies to elucidate how foods affect body weight, cholesterol, blood pressure, diabetes, and chronic pain. Some of our studies have been very influential. In 2003, the National Institutes of Health funded us to test a new dietary approach to type 2 diabetes that turned out to be the most powerful program of its kind ever developed. Many people are using it to improve their diabetes and sometimes even make it go away.

We worked with GEICO—the insurance company—to see how a nutrition program might work in the workplace, finding that simple diet changes can revolutionize the health of employees. In 2015, the U.S. government cited our research work as strong evidence for recommending plant-based diets in the Dietary Guidelines for Americans.

In the course of our studies, I have noticed an odd phenomenon. A surprising number of people whose health dramatically improved from dietary changes reported that, despite all their health improvements, they still found themselves having a hankering for cheese. Not ice cream, not yogurt, not chocolate milk, but specifically cheese. Even when cheese had been a huge contributor to their health problems, their cravings made it hard to tear themselves away.

After hearing this over and over, I began to study cheese's effects on our health and to investigate why it has such a surprisingly strong attraction. This book shares what I've found. I hope you find it enlightening, fun, encouraging, and powerful. And I hope you will share the power of what you are about to learn with everyone you know. I wish you the very best of health.

CHAPTER 1

The Ultimate Processed Food

Fugu is the world's second-strangest food. Fugu is the Japanese word for the meat of the puffer fish, that small creature who, when threatened, turns himself into a spike-covered balloon. Puffer fish have more than spikes; they also harbor deadly tetrodotoxin. One bite contains enough poison to paralyze your diaphragm and arrest your breathing.

The possibility of death by suffocation has not stopped adventurous diners from wanting to taste it. And Japanese chefs have been willing to dedicate three or more years of their lives to learning the fine art of separating the poisonous and non-poisonous puffer fish parts in order to be legally allowed to serve it.

You really have to wonder, how did this start? What courageous adventurers were willing to experiment, Russian roulette–style, with various puffer fish organs until they got it right?

Well, the puffer fish has nothing on Camembert. Cheese

is easily the world's strangest food, and the most improbable. Mother Nature never imagined anything like this.

First of all, one of our human forebears had to *want* to take milk from another species. It apparently took two and a half million years of human existence before that idea popped into someone's head. Then he or she had to figure out how to make an animal stand still long enough to extract her milk. That, too, was a challenge, when you consider the size of the animals involved and the fact that very few would be lactating at the appropriate time. And since animals produce milk only for a limited period of time after giving birth, our prehistoric food pioneer would have had to sort out how to keep milk flowing.

Then he or she had to mix the milk with bacteria to ferment it, and then combine it with enzymes hidden in the lining of the fourth stomach of a calf.

Finally, people had to *like* the gooey result—which was not a foregone conclusion, given that the smell of cheese is the smell of bacterial decomposition. In fact, the brevibacteria used to produce Muenster, Limburger, and several other common cheeses are the very germs responsible for the stench of unwashed human feet.

What are the odds? Makes fugu sound easy.

Indeed, cheese was not exactly an overnight sensation. There was not a single cheese factory in the U.S. until 1851, and it was not until 1935 that the average American ate even 5 pounds of it per year. But eventually it found its way into our hearts.

Into our coronary arteries, to be more precise. And into our thighs and hips, and spilling onto our medical charts. The health problems cheese causes are more subtle and protracted than puffer fish poisoning, but they are extremely common. So much so that most people assume they are just part of life.

In this chapter, we'll take a look at this odd, familiar, smelly, and loved product; how cheese makers turn a pail of milk into a block of cheese; and how a product of bacterial decomposition becomes hard to resist. In later chapters, we will see what happens when you swallow it.

Making Cheese

Cheese making is not without some theoretical advantages. Anyone who drinks milk knows that it does not stay fresh very long; turning it into cheese preserves it. Along the way, cheese concentrates milk's fat, protein, and calories. It also makes it a lot more portable.

Cheese also eliminates lactose, the milk sugar that is indigestible for many people. Nursing babies can digest lactose and use it for energy. But after the age of weaning, the enzymes that digest lactose start to disappear and, without them, milk causes cramps and diarrhea. Although many people—especially whites—carry a genetic mutation that makes those enzymes persist longer, the majority of adults are lactose-intolerant. But when milk is turned into cheese, that indigestible lactose is mostly removed.

To see how cheese is made, let's take a trip to the tiny town of Theresa, Wisconsin, northwest of Milwaukee. A little factory on Henni Street has been cranking out cheese since 1900. In 1905, John Widmer arrived in the U.S. from Switzerland, learned the cheese-making craft, and eventually took over the factory. It has stayed in the Widmer family ever since.

As you arrive in Theresa, you realize that you saw surprisingly few cows along the country roads. Obviously, the number-one cheese-producing state would need lots and lots of cows, but the fields were empty, for the most part. Where they are is something we'll touch on in Chapter 7.

Nonetheless, a huge milk shipment arrives at the Widmer's Cheese Cellars factory early each morning and is poured into two large vats, each about twenty feet long and three feet deep. It takes more than a gallon of milk to make a pound of Cheddar.

Because milk comes from a living, breathing animal, its chemical makeup varies from batch to batch, and that affects the taste or texture of the cheese. So cheese producers can head off problems by *standardizing* the milk—adding cream, skim milk, or skim milk powder, as the case may be, to keep the fat and protein content uniform from batch to batch.

They can also adjust the color. Cheese's orange color comes, in part, from traces of beta-carotene in milk—the same beta-carotene that gives an orange color to carrots and sweet potatoes. It is too dilute to be seen in milk, but it becomes visible as milk fat is concentrated in the cheese-making process. Widmer's and other cheese makers can legally intensify the color with *annatto*, a tree extract from Latin America and the Caribbean.

Goats, sheep, and water buffalos do not secrete beta-carotene into their milk as cows do, so their cheese is white. To make cow's milk mozzarella look white, some manufacturers add titanium dioxide or peroxides. Dunkin' Donuts used the same trick to make its powdered sugar extra white—until consumer complaints led to its removal.

Where Does Milk Come From?

All mammalian species make milk, but few will ever be recruited for cheese. Milk from horses and camels does not coagulate properly, and most other mammals are not the right size or temperament for the demands of the dairy industry. Most are too small to produce much milk, and some are too large and dangerous.

Roughly nine million cows are on U.S. dairy farms at any given time, a number that is gradually falling as breeders and pharmaceutical manufacturers find ways to push each cow to produce more milk. Holsteins—the common black-and-white cows you see in pictures—each produce more than 2,800 gallons (11,000 liters) per year. Occasionally, dairy farmers use Jerseys (light brown with white patches) and, less commonly, Brown Swiss, Ayrshires, Guernseys, and other breeds whose milk is less plentiful but is higher in fat and protein.

Italian mozzarella comes from the milk of water buffalos. Goats and sheep make high-fat, high-protein, high-cholesterol milk used for feta and other popular European cheeses.

In the United States, nearly all milk is pasteurized—that is, it is briefly heated to knock out disease-causing bacteria. Some cheese enthusiasts prefer unpasteurized "raw milk" cheeses, but these products cannot be sold in interstate commerce in the United States.

Bring on the Bugs

With the vats now filled like milky wading pools, the next step is to add bacterial cultures. The bacteria ferment the milk sugar, *lactose*, to produce lactic acid, which contributes to the flavor of cheese.

What kind of bacteria? For a mild product, cheese makers use strains that produce lactic acid and not much else. For other varieties, they add cultures that produce various flavors and perhaps bubbles (to make holes). And they might eventually add molds and yeast, adding scents and tastes of their own.

Some bacteria are particularly stinky. Take *brevibacteria*, for example. This bacterial genus is ubiquitous. They are all over your skin and down your socks. If you haven't washed your feet in a while, it's those overgrowing brevibacteria that make people open the windows.

Brevibacteria are used to produce Muenster, Limburger, and several other cheeses, as we saw earlier. If these cheeses smell like unwashed feet, it's because you're smelling precisely the same thing.

Some cheese cultures include *Staphylococcus epidermidis*, one of the bacterial species responsible for human B.O. If you're hungry for details, the bacteria produce isovaleric acid (3-methylbutanoic acid), which imparts a characteristic odor to the human armpit and to some strong cheeses.

One of the compounds often produced during cheese making—butyric acid—is also produced when your stomach acid digests food, which is why, to many people, Parmesan has a faint odor of vomit.

As the cheese-making process proceeds, milk fats and proteins break down into a wide variety of chemical products, one of which is *skatole*. If you notice a slight off-odor (let's face it, cheese does not smell like roses), that is because skatole is also responsible for part of the odor of human feces (it is produced from tryptophan in the human intestine). The U.S. military has also used skatole for its nonlethal "stinkbomb" "malodorant weaponry" designed to temporarily incapacitate the enemy. But you can get it without a military contract. It is in ordinary cheese.

The human nose is exquisitely sensitive to bacterial decomposition, alerting us to food that has gone bad as well as to fecal contamination and other unclean things. But it is precisely the scents of decomposing food, unwashed feet, B.O., and human waste that end up in cheese.

Calves' Stomachs or Genetic Engineering?

Okay, our milk is standardized, pasteurized, and color-adjusted, and bacteria have been busily fermenting it. Now, it's time to coagulate it, turning fluid milk into solid curd. To do this, cheese makers add *rennet*—enzymes that break apart milk proteins and fats. Traditionally, rennet was taken from calves' stomachs, and Widmer's still uses this source. The liquefied calf extract looks a bit like tea as it is poured into the mix.

Most cheese makers use genetically engineered rennet. In 1990, the U.S. Food and Drug Administration approved the process in which enzyme-producing genes are inserted into bacteria and fungi, which, in turn, produce rennet. And some cheeses are coagulated without rennet, using plant extracts or—in the case of cream cheese, paneer, and other soft cheeses—citric acid, vinegar, and similar acids.

Rennet causes the curds to form, and the watery *whey* is then drained off. And that presents a new challenge, especially for large-scale cheese makers. What do you do with all that useless whey? Cheese factories put out tons of it, and it will take quite a landfill to handle that load of cheese factory waste.

As it happens, the dairy industry found a market for whey. Packed in a tub, whey protein is heavily promoted to body builders who can be induced to pay top dollar in hopes that it will pump up their muscles.

Forming and Salting

Time to pour the curds into a form—a round one to produce a wheel, a rectangular one to produce a block. These *forms* have also produced names for cheese: In Italian it is *formaggio*, in French *fromage*.

To make brick cheese—a Wisconsin original invented in 1877—Widmer's cheese makers pile on actual bricks, squeezing out the last bits of water and whey protein. And, yes, they use the same bricks that Granddad used.

Along the way, salt is added to stop bacterial growth and add flavor. As we will see in the next chapter, a surprising amount of salt ends up in every slice of cheese you'll find at the store.

Widmer's cheese blocks then go into the curing room, where warm, humid conditions encourage bacterial growth. Over the next week, the surface will be washed daily with bacteria, then the bricks are wrapped in parchment and foil for sale.

Human Cheese?

You might be wondering if it is possible to make cheese from human milk. The answer is no—at least, not very well. It is too low in the casein protein that is abundant in cow's milk, and does not coagulate especially well. But that has not stopped people from trying. At Klee Brasserie in New York, *Iron Chef* champion Daniel Angerer made cheese from a 50:50 mixture of cow's milk and his wife's breast milk before the New York Health Department made him stop.

At a New York art gallery, art student Miriam Simun offered three varieties of cheese made from milk donated by breast-feeding mothers. It was not a hit. A writer for the *Village Voice* wrote, "There is something fundamentally disgusting about it...No one knows what the effect of human breast milk on adults will be. The milk contains a complex mixture of nutrients, hormones, and antibodies formulated by Mother Nature not for adults, but for the youngest babies."

Which raises the obvious question: If it is so disgusting to make cheese from human milk, is cow's milk any better? After all, it was produced in the body of a cow for her baby, not for humans of any age. Does it affect health, too?

I'm glad you asked. Stay tuned. We'll tackle exactly that question in due course.

Endless Varieties

There are, of course, countless varieties of cheese that differ from each other based on the animal species they come from, the bacterial cultures used, the aging process, and other factors.

Cottage cheese and cream cheese are coagulated with acid, using little or no rennet. They retain a bit of lactose sugar and are not aged, which is why their flavors are mild.

Ricotta (Italian for "recooked") is made from whey, rather than casein.

Feta is traditionally made from sheep's milk or a combination of sheep's and goat's milk.

Although mozzarella traditionally comes from the milk of water buffalos, as we saw above, in the United States it is made from cow's milk. Thanks to its use on pizza, it has overtaken Cheddar as the number-one cheese in America.

Camembert and Brie, from northern France, are made with bacteria, mold, and yeast that contribute their own smells and flavors—objectionable to some, addictive to others. Only one small Camembert factory remains in the village of Camembert. Fromagerie Durand is happy to show you its cows standing in thick manure and the process of turning their milk into cheese.

Roquefort, Gorgonzola, and Stilton have mold introduced into their interiors. Roquefort is made with sheep's milk, Gorgonzola and Stilton with cow's milk.

Emmental (or Emmentaler), from Switzerland, is famous for its holes ("eyes"), which are the result of bacterial cultures producing carbon dioxide gas.

In medieval times, Edam's red outer color came from turnsole dye, according to Michael Tunick, a U.S. Department of Agriculture cheese scientist. Rags soaked with dye were hung over pans of urine. The urine's ammonia heightened the color of the dye, which was then rubbed onto the cheese. Today, the cheese's color comes from a red wax coating.

Limburger, born in what is now a region of Belgium, Germany, and the Netherlands, is famous for its pungent smell. Steve, who is one of my colleagues at the Physicians Committee, recalled his Limburger experiences, which started during a teenage summer job. He handled maintenance duties at a summer camp for high school kids at Lake Como, Pennsylvania, mowing the lawns, fixing broken light switches, and basically keeping the place running. One day, he was asked to take one of the camp administrators for a ride into town.

Steve hopped in the driver's seat. The camp administrator buckled into the passenger seat, and the two set off. A few minutes later, a death-like smell filled the car. Only later did they find out that Steve's shop boss, an inveterate practical joker, had put a block of Limburger on Steve's exhaust manifold.

Not long thereafter, Steve decided to pledge to a college fraternity in Bloomsburg, Pennsylvania. That meant hazing: nineteen days and twenty nights of physical and mental tests and various humiliating and sometimes dangerous experiences. And most memorable of all was *Cheese Night*. The young would-be frat members lined up outside the frat house in front of a table stacked high with—you guessed it—Limburger. The challenge: Eat it. Eat it until you throw up! Which, in Steve's case, was not long.

Cheddar is the bestselling cheese outside the U.S. and is

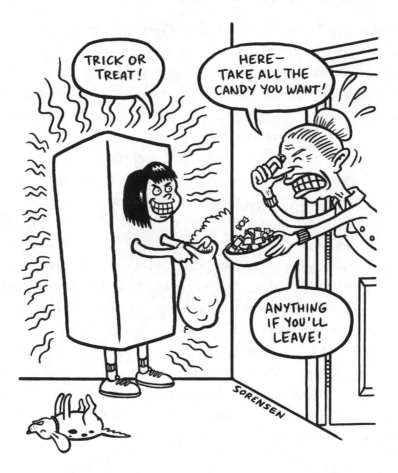

**AMANDA'S LIMBURGER CHEESE COSTUME
PAID OFF HANDSOMELY.**

made with a process called *cheddaring*. Widmer's will gladly show you how they do it. But cheddaring did not begin in Wisconsin. It began in Cheddar.

In Somerset, a two-hour drive west of London, the village of Cheddar has three schools, a supermarket, and a long string of stores catering to tourists, along with a deep, picturesque gorge and huge caves. That's where, a thousand years ago, the world's favorite cheese was born. Just one cheese factory remains today.

But the folks at the Cheddar Gorge Cheese Company will show you the process that starts anew each morning.

Similarly to the production of other cheeses, milk goes into a huge vat and is briefly heated. In go the bacterial cultures, followed by rennet to coagulate the milk into a semi-solid mass. The nascent cheese is then cut, allowing the whey to rise to the surface. The mixture is heated again, and the bacterial fermentation process swings into high gear, creating lactic acid. The watery whey mixture—containing protein and sugar—is then drained off to be fed to pigs.

The curds are shoveled onto a cooling table, and this is where cheddaring begins. Big slabs of curd are cut, turned, and stacked one on top of the other. The process is repeated over and over, allowing more whey to be drained away as the curd firms up.

The cheese makers add salt—lots of it—then shred the slabs and pour them into large paint can–sized steel molds and press them, squeezing out more whey. The cheese is then removed from the molds, scalded in water for a smooth outer surface, then put back into the molds to be pressed again, and then again—three times in all. Eventually the cheese is ready to be aged and sold.

Leaping Maggots

A certain species of fly, *Piophila casei*, is especially fond of decomposing protein, like corpses and cheese. In Sardinia and Corsica, cheese makers encourage the flies to lay their eggs on a sheep's milk cheese called *Pecorino*. As the maggots hatch, they digest the cheese, producing a liquefied mass called *casu marzu* ("rotten cheese"). Diners spread it—maggots and all—on flatbread, then hold their hands over the sandwich to avoid being struck by the leaping larvae. They wash it down with red wine.

Process Cheese

Enough about Cheddar, feta, Camembert, and maggots. What about good old American *process cheese*? You can thank James L. Kraft for it. In 1916, the Kraft Foods founder patented a method for blending old, unsold cheese with younger cheese and adding various ingredients to improve its flavor, color, texture, and shelf-life. (And, yes, it's called "process cheese," even though most people now call it "processed.")

Today, there are many variants, each with its own legal name. But there is one particularly important variety, which I discovered as a college student on a sightseeing trip to Mexico. Stopping into a local restaurant just south of the border, we ordered cheese tostadas—crisp tortillas covered with a spiced cheese topping.

"This is delicious," I said to the server. "What is it?" What Mexican secret tradition was in this amazing dish? I was envisioning some magically prepared cheese carefully spiced to perfection.

"It's Velveeta," he said.

Yes, Velveeta.

That quintessential American food was invented by Emil Frey, a Swiss cheese maker who went to work for the Monroe Cheese Company in New York. He had already created an American version of Limburger, called *Liederkranz*, and, in 1918, he combined leftover and broken bits of cheese with whey and other ingredients to make a smooth, meltable product. He launched the Velveeta Cheese Company in 1923, and four years later, it was gobbled up by Kraft Foods.

Today, Velveeta is made with milk, whey protein, milk fat, food starch, and other ingredients, along with annatto and apocarotenal for color.

And Now the Problems Start

Cheese is tasty, in an old-socks kind of way. Lots of people love it. So, apart from the occasional leaping maggot, what harm could it do? Well, have a look at what the cheese-making process actually does:

- First, it concentrates calories. A cup of milk has 149 calories; a cup of melted Cheddar has close to a thousand (986, to be exact). If you're thinking metric, 200 grams of milk has 122 calories; 200 grams of Cheddar has 808.
- Second, it concentrates dairy proteins, particularly casein. For some people, these proteins trigger respiratory symptoms, migraines, arthritis, skin conditions, and other problems.
- Third, it concentrates cholesterol and saturated fat, the "bad fat" that raises cholesterol levels and increases the risk of heart disease and Alzheimer's disease.
- As if all that were not enough, there is enough salt in cheese to contribute to high blood pressure. Along with it, cheese contains a variety of chemicals, from hormones to opiates, that makes it a product like no other.

All of which makes an important point: Cheese is a heavily processed food. If you look askance at spaghetti or bread because they are *processed*, that is, they are made from grains that are—gasp—*ground up*, think for a minute about cheese. Cheese is the ultimate processed glop.

Cheese started life as grass. The protein, calcium, and other nutrients in those blades of grass went down the hatch of a cow. Passing through the cow's stomachs and digestive tract, those nutrients were transformed by stomach acid and various enzymes and eventually found their way into the cow's body and eventually into the milk. The milk was then pasteurized, fermented by bacteria, coagulated with enzymes, separated into solids, salted, and aged, during which time it was further metabolized by bacteria or other germs. Later, it might be added to a pizza or a casserole, only to be baked and salted again. It's hard to find a more heavily processed product.

The Yellow Tsunami

In 1909, the U.S. Department of Agriculture began tracking American eating habits. In that year, the average American ate less than 4 pounds of cheese *in a year* (3.8 pounds, to be exact). Cheese was really a European product back in those days. It was not what we ate in Peoria, and it had no effect on the American waistline.

But things changed. In the 1960s, fast-food chains cropped up like weeds, and there was not a burger that a grill cook couldn't slap a slice of cheese on. After these first yellow ripples, the tsunami arrived. It was called pizza.

Pizza in restaurants, schools, and grocery freezers brought tons of cheese to American plates. Unlike a traditional Italian pizza that uses a sprinkling of cheese as a flavoring (or sometimes no cheese at all), American pizzas are essentially delivery vehicles for ever-deeper layers of gooey cheese. By 2013, the average American's annual cheese intake had climbed from less than four pounds in 1909 to more than 33 pounds. That's roughly 30 pounds of extra cheese this year, next year, and the year after that.

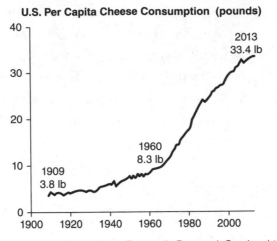

Source: U.S. Department of Agriculture, Economic Research Service, http://ers.usda
.gov/data-products/food-availability-(per-capita)-data-system/.aspx#26705. Accessed
November 14, 2015.

What does 30 extra pounds of cheese mean, measured in calories? Take a guess.

Maybe a thousand? No, there are more calories than that in just *one* pound of cheese.

Maybe ten thousand? Twenty thousand? Actually, the 30 pounds of cheese that the average American has added to his or her annual diet hold *55,000 calories*. You could drink a can of Coke every day and not get to 55,000 calories. That's 55,000 extra calories this year, the same again next year, and the same every year, if not more. In the next chapter, we will see exactly how cheese makes us fat, but by now you're already starting to get a sense of why it packs on the pounds.

Who is making all this stuff? The United States is. America is, by far, the world's leading cheese producer, with Germany a distant second and France in third place.[1] But when it comes to *exports*, France and Germany are numbers one and two. The U.S. is not even in the top ten. We eat it all ourselves.

In the chapters that follow, we will look at how this peculiar, processed, fatty invention affects our waistline, the surprising ways it triggers health problems, and why it keeps us hooked. And we will look at how to tackle these problems, with an especially detailed look at how to enjoy truly delicious food and get the best of health in the bargain.

CHAPTER 2

More Calories Than Coke, More Salt Than Potato Chips: What Cheese Does to Your Waistline

In 1966, Joey Vento opened Geno's Steaks at the corner of Ninth and Passyunk, and tourists flock there to taste the food that *is* Philadelphia. Geno's cooks up rib eye steak and serves it on bread baked on-site. And what kind of cheese goes on a cheesesteak? Not the kind of people to put on airs, Geno's says on its website, "Well it's cheese. You can never really go wrong with cheese." In the kitchen, you'll find American, provolone, and Cheez Whiz, which go on the sandwich with a handful of onions.

The crowds were predictable. And so, perhaps, was what happened to Joey. In 2010, he was diagnosed with colon cancer, and in the following year he was killed by a heart attack.

Joey had named his son Geno after the restaurant. Growing up in the business, young Geno developed a taste for the kinds of foods the restaurant sold and the not-so-different foods served at home. "I loved cheese fries," Geno said. "They were my happy food. And pizza, mozzarella sticks, and mac and cheese."

It didn't help that he often found himself in the spotlight at public events. As the son of an iconic and wildly successful restaurateur, Geno was expected to be the fun, entertaining center of attention—and to eat whatever was served. It is still true today. Geno is a well-known philanthropist, and that means he is often called to charity dinners where he has to be "on" and has to eat.

By the time he reached high school, Geno weighed 240 pounds. And he was eager to tackle the problem. He tried Nutrisystem, Weight Watchers, Jenny Craig, diet pills, and every other weight-loss method he could find. His father offered his own ideas: "Just shut your mouth. Exercise more."

But he found there was also an addictive side to food. "I can be good from morning through dinner. But between dinner and bedtime is my danger zone. The Devil comes out. If I'm hanging out with friends, my vice is food."

Eventually, Geno carried 360 pounds on his five-foot, eight-inch frame. At age forty, he was diagnosed with prediabetes and sleep apnea—an obesity-related disorder.

After his father's death, Geno decided to get serious. He had weight-loss surgery and eventually he lost more than 100 pounds.

Yes, It Matters

How much difference can cheese really make? Let's say I add a bit of cheese to my salad every day. Or maybe I top my pizza with a bit more mozzarella. Will I gain weight? Or what if, like in Geno's family, cheese is a big part of our daily routine?

Those were the kinds of questions a team of New Zealand scientists asked in a 2014 research study.[1] They went down this road because some doctors and dietitians encourage patients to include dairy products in their diets (as do restaurants and cheese manufacturers, needless to say). So the question was: If people follow that advice, what happens?

The researchers asked volunteers to make a point of including cheese and similar dairy products in their diets—two or three servings a day. So that meant having a glass of milk instead of soda, or adding a slice of cheese to a burger.

You might imagine that, if you're adding a bit of cheese, you're likely to compensate by eating less of something else, so your weight ought to stay about the same. After all, if I have a grilled cheese sandwich instead of peanut butter and jelly, what's the difference? And if there's extra mozzarella on my salad, I'm going to fill up sooner and set down my fork before I've overdone it. My weight shouldn't change, right? Well, that's not what happened. After a month, the people who added dairy products gained a bit of weight. The amount was small—about a pound in a month's time, on average. That sounds pretty benign, doesn't it—one pound per month? Except that there are twelve months in a year.

For perspective, the average American adult puts on about a pound and a half of weight *per year.* That works out to 15 pounds per decade, 30 pounds over twenty years, and so on. Some people gain more than that, of course, and others don't gain weight at all. But those numbers are the averages. So if a food makes you gain *an extra pound per month*, as these research participants were doing, you are actually gaining weight much more rapidly than the average person.

Other research studies have shown the same thing. Even though adding more cheese to your diet ought to mean you will compensate by eating less of something else, the scale shows a real difference. A 2013 meta-analysis combined the results of ten prior studies, and even though 60 percent of the studies were funded by the dairy industry, the verdict was clear. Slowly but surely, cheese pads your waistline, fills out your cheeks, and shows up on the scale.[2]

At Harvard University, researchers have studied the diets of doctors, nurses, and other health professionals for decades. The idea is that these health-conscious, well-educated people ought to be accurate at reporting what they eat and in describing whatever health problems might result. In 2015, the researchers looked specifically at cheese and similar foods and, yes, the more cheese people ate, the more weight they gained.[3]

Researchers at Loma Linda University in California looked at this question in another way. Zeroing in on vegetarians, they found that some ate cheese and other dairy products, while others did not. The researchers measured everyone's height and weight and calculated their BMI—that is, their body mass index (your BMI is essentially your weight adjusted for how tall you are; a healthy BMI is below 25).

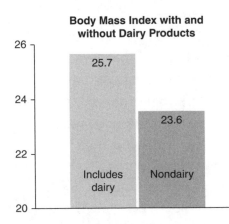

Body Mass Index with and without Dairy Products

Source: Tonstad S., et al. *Diabetes Care*: 2009; 32:791–96.

For those who skipped cheese and other dairy products, the average BMI was a healthy 23.6. But those who had a taste for grilled cheese or cheesy lasagna or other dairy-based foods had an average BMI of 25.7.

That works out to a 15-pound weight difference, on average, between those who include cheese and other dairy products and those who avoid them.

So, is cheese fattening? In a word, yes. Or, in six words: There is no question about it. People who eat cheese tend to have weight problems, and controlled research studies clearly show the weight-gain effect.

Okay, But Why?

If you're wondering how cheese packs on the pounds, here is what puts the chubby in Cheddar:

Cheese has lots of calories. To state the obvious, cheese has calories—a lot of them. Remember, milk is nature's food for fattening a calf, and that means the cow packs a lot of calories into it. And as we saw in Chapter 1, the process of cheese making takes the calories in milk and concentrates them even more.

We touched on the numbers in the last chapter. Let's take a closer look: If we were to fill a measuring cup with whole milk, it would end up with 149 calories. That's plenty—more than a can of Coke. Now, let's fill the same cup with melted Cheddar. It turns out to be almost seven times higher, at 986 calories per cup. Not that most people would use that much cheese, but you get the idea: Cheese is concentrated calories. Think about it melted over a pizza, over a burger, inside an omelet—and gradually expanding your waistline.

Now let's look at typical serving sizes. For comparison, a can of Coke has 140 calories. If you were to make a grilled cheese sandwich with 2 ounces of process cheese, you'd get 170 calories from the cheese alone. Two ounces of Brie have about 190 calories. And 2 ounces of Cheddar have about 230.

Of course, you can buy Coke Zero and get zero calories, more or less. But there is no Cheddar Zero, Brie Zero, Velveeta Zero, or any other Cheese Zero.

And there is more to it. The calories in cheese are often *added* calories. When a slice of cheese is added to a hamburger, nothing is taken away. Piled higher on a pizza, nothing is removed to compensate for those extra calories. The cheese industry is well aware of this. As we will see in Chapter 8, people can be pushed to eat more and more of it, putting more money in cheese makers' cash registers and more calories than ever onto our plates.

Those calories come from fat. It's not just that cheese has calories. Its calories come mostly from fat, and fat calories are a particular problem.

Here's why: Fat that you eat adds easily to your body fat. You swallow it, tiny particles of fat enter your bloodstream, and with relatively little change they can pack into your fat cells.

Compare that to eating bread. During digestion, the starch in bread releases glucose—simple sugar—into your bloodstream. That sugar does not look anything like fat, and it will not end up in your body fat, for the most part. Rather, your body uses it for power. Glucose fuels your movements, powers your brain, maintains your body temperature, and keeps your other basic body functions running, as opposed to turning into fat.

If you were to overindulge a bit on bread, your body still does not want to make fat. Rather, it stores excess glucose as *glycogen*—molecules that act like spare batteries in your muscles and liver.

If you were to keep overeating carbohydrate-rich foods— more than you need for basic energy and more than you can store as glycogen—your body would eventually convert the sugar molecules from that unneeded carbohydrate into fat. But turning sugar into fat is not especially easy for the body to do. The process of turning sugar into fat uses up almost a quarter of its calories.

So while it is possible for your body to turn bread or sugar into fat, it is not easy, and a lot of calories are lost in the process. It is much easier for your body to turn cheese fat or other fats into body fat.

Fat can slow your metabolism. It gets worse. Not only does fat in foods get stored as body fat. It also packs into your muscle cells, and there, it can interfere with your metabolism.

You have probably heard that your muscles are calorie burners; you want to preserve your muscle mass so that you can burn calories. That's true enough. Inside your muscle cells are microscopic burners called *mitochondria*. They power your cells.

However, when you eat fatty foods, some of that fat works its way into your muscle cells. And as it builds up, it interferes with the cells' ability to produce mitochondria, gradually reducing the number of mitochondria in your cells. In the process, fatty foods can slow your metabolism.

Imagine, if you will, a gas stove. Sitting on one of the burners is a pot filled with melted cheese. The cheese is bubbling up and spattering onto the stove. Some of it is melting down the side of the pot and dripping onto the burner. At first, it sputters and burns, but when more and more of it dribbles onto the burner, it puts the flame out. In a way, that is what happens in your body. Fatty foods interfere with your microscopic burners.

It happens fast. Scientists in Baton Rouge, Louisiana, asked ten healthy men to follow a high-fat diet as part of an experiment. Taking muscle biopsies, the researchers found that it takes only three days for fatty foods to slow down the genes that produce mitochondria. The long-term result of this process is that it becomes harder and harder to burn fat.[4] It appears that *saturated* fats (prevalent in cheese and meat) are worse in this regard than *unsaturated* fats (found in vegetable oils).[5]

Researchers at Virginia Tech made a similar observation. Their research kitchen cooked up fatty meals (drawing 55 percent of their calories from fat, compared with around 30 to 35 percent, which is average for Americans), and the researchers asked volunteers to eat these fatty foods for five days straight. The volunteers came in every morning for breakfast and picked up their meals for the rest of the day. After five days, the researchers took tiny samples of the participants' muscle cells, finding that, yes, they were less able to metabolize calories.[6] Their burners were not working so well anymore.

It might sound surprising that fatty foods can slow down metabolism. But think about it. Our bodies were *designed*, if I can use that word, millions of years ago, when famine was a very real threat. Back then, if you were to come across a particularly abundant food source, your body was eager to store as many calories as possible, in case food might be in short supply later on. Now, if your mitochondria were to just keep on burning calories full blast, there would not be much left to store. So your body turns down its mitochondrial production, burning calories more slowly, so you can save some fat in your cells.

That was great back then. Nowadays, we don't want to store fat; we'd like to shed it. But our bodies are pre-programmed, and fatty foods still slow our metabolisms today, just as they did in the distant past.

Sodium adds water weight. Cheese is loaded with sodium—that is, salt. It is added as a preservative and flavoring. But salt increases your water weight, and the explanation for this is not so mysterious.

Sodium in foods is rapidly absorbed into your bloodstream and tends to hold water, both in your blood and in your body tissues. That makes you feel heavy and bloated, and it shows up as a couple of extra pounds on the scale. And, of course, because salt makes foods extra palatable, we sometimes dig in a bit more than we otherwise would. More on that in the next chapter. But the point for now is that salty foods tend to increase water weight.

Is there really a lot of salt in cheese? Well, have a look. For comparison, a 2-ounce pack of potato chips has about 330 milligrams of sodium. A 2-ounce serving of Cheddar or Muenster has more than 350. A similar serving of Edam has more than 500, and 2 ounces of Velveeta have—hold on to your blood pressure—*more than 800 milligrams* of sodium.

People looking to limit salt may not think of cheese as a high-sodium food, but it is right near the top of the list. When you throw out the cheese and other salty foods, that water weight quickly disappears, and you can see the difference on your scale.

What Cheese Doesn't Have

So calories, fat, and sodium are a recipe for weight gain. But there is one thing that cheese *doesn't* have.

Fiber is plant roughage. There is a lot of it in beans, vegetables, fruits, and whole grains. What makes it special is that it is filling but has essentially no calories. Fiber makes you feel full, so you push away from the table and feel satisfied without overdoing it.

Cheese is not a plant, so it has zero fiber. When you bite into a slice of cheese, there is nothing between you and every last calorie it holds. That means you can swallow a lot of calories before you feel even close to full.

One more thing: We've hinted that cheese is addictive, and we will have much more to say about this in the next chapter. But addictive foods don't just keep us hooked. Sometimes they stimulate more eating. In other words, you are not just getting a daily "fix" from cheese. You're overdoing it—getting more calories than you need and more than your body can manage.

Can Feta Make You Fat?

If fatty cheeses are fattening, what about feta? Isn't it more natural? You be the judge: Using a 140-calorie Coke for comparison, 2 ounces of feta weigh in at 150 calories, with 12 grams of fat and an enormous 520 milligrams of sodium. And, like all cheeses, not a speck of fiber.

You will find some low-fat cheeses. If Kraft Shredded Low-Moisture Part-Skim Mozzarella with Added Calcium whets your appetite, 2 ounces bring you 140 calories, 9 grams of fat, and 360 milligrams of sodium. And there is a fat-free version with 90 calories and—gulp—560 milligrams of sodium. But not surprisingly, studies show that adding low-fat dairy products tends to cause weight gain, too.[7] It's a load of unnecessary calories, with no fiber at all. These products provide no nutritional advantages and just contribute to weight gain.

Gut Bacteria

It is easy to understand why cheese would contribute to weight problems. It is loaded with calories that were intended for a growing calf. Its fat adds easily to body fat, without much biochemical conversion. Plus, it can slow your metabolism just like other fatty foods, it is missing the fiber you need to control your appetite, its sodium adds insult to injury in the form of water weight, and its addictive effect stimulates you to eat more.

There might be other reasons, too. Researchers have found that fatty foods make your digestive tract wall more permeable, so that calorie-packed molecules can slip through and pass into your bloodstream.[8]

Here is what they are suggesting: Normally, your digestive tract is choosy about what it allows to pass into your bloodstream. Not everything you eat is going to pass from your intestinal tract into your blood. But it appears that certain foods can change that. Researchers believe that fatty foods encourage the growth of intestinal bacteria that not only release more calories from otherwise indigestible foods, but can also foster their passage into the bloodstream. This is a hot area of research, so stay tuned.

Putting It to the Test

In our research center, we have tested the effects of getting away from cheese and other animal products.[9] In one study, our participants were women who had been struggling with weight problems for years. Over fourteen weeks, we took cheese and all other animal products out of their diets. The rules were (1) avoid animal products and (2) minimize added oils. We did not ask them to count calories or limit carbohydrates or portion sizes. Just the opposite; they were free to eat all the pancakes with maple syrup they wanted. But cheesy omelets and bacon were out. Veggie burgers were okay, but the meat varieties were out. Spaghetti could be topped with tomatoes, wild mushrooms, artichoke hearts, and fresh basil, but not Alfredo sauce. We also asked everyone to keep their exercise routines constant, so we could zero in on what the diet changes were doing.

After fourteen weeks, everyone stood on the scale. The average person had lost 13 pounds. Considering they had not been counting calories or limiting portions, that was impressive. We then followed our participants over the next twelve months, finding that they were slimmer at one year than at the beginning of the study. We followed them for an additional year, and, yes, they were slimmer at two years than at one year. In other words, weight loss was essentially a one-way street.

How does this happen? Why did they lose weight? The answer is not hard to find. Without those fatty foods, their meals had fewer calories. And with plenty of high-fiber vegetables, fruits, whole grains, and beans, their meals were more filling. That's the first part of the explanation.

But there was more to it. Their metabolisms were getting back to normal.

Before the study began, many of our participants said they felt that their metabolisms had slowed over time. "When I was sixteen, I could eat anything," one said. "But now, I just look at food, and I gain weight!"

So we actually measured the participants' metabolic rates. Each participant lay down on an examination table, and with a special monitoring device, we tracked how much oxygen she took in and how much carbon dioxide she exhaled, and some simple arithmetic gave us the number of calories she was burning minute by minute.

After fourteen weeks on the animal product–free diet, we found that the average participant's after-meal metabolism had increased by 16 percent. That's a small change, but over time it contributes to the calorie burn that can help trim away pounds.

What we believe happened was that their mitochondria were rebounding, just as we saw earlier. That means a better metabolism.

So why does getting away from cheese and similar products lead to impressive weight loss? First, you are avoiding cheese's mother lode of calories. Second, you're getting lots of fiber to fill you up. And third, your after-meal metabolism is ramped up a notch.

We have done similar studies with hundreds of men and women, and have found powerful weight loss in every study. Working with GEICO—the insurance company—we invited company employees in ten different cities to join a program offering healthy foods at work for eighteen weeks.[10] They were free to eat as much as they wanted, but everything they chose was healthy—free of animal products and low in fat. Even though we asked everyone not to cut calories and not to change their exercise habits, the average person lost weight. In related studies, people with diabetes, high cholesterol, high blood pressure, arthritis, or migraines have often found that these conditions improve dramatically, too. More on those topics in Chapters 5 and 6.

The take-home message is that, yes, cheese really is fattening. Getting it and other fatty foods out of your diet can trim away the pounds, improve your health in many ways, and even help your metabolism.

New Power for Health

It is time to celebrate. You now have knowledge that has eluded many other people. And it is knowledge you can put to work right now.

To see the importance of this, flash back to November 12, 2015. The *New York Times* ran a story entitled "Obesity Rises Despite All Efforts to Fight It, U.S. Health Officials Say." The article said, "Despite years of efforts to reduce obesity in America, including a major push by Michelle Obama, federal health officials reported Thursday that the share of Americans who were obese had not declined in recent years, and had edged up slightly."

It was sad, but true. In 2003 and 2004, 32 percent of American adults were obese. Ten years later, the number was not one bit better. It was actually up to 38 percent. Marion Nestle, of New York University, said, "Everybody was hoping that with the decline in sugar and soda consumption, that we'd start seeing a leveling off of adult obesity." Indeed, sugar consumption had dropped—about 15 percent since the late 1990s. But waistlines were bigger than ever, and health authorities were left wringing their hands.

If you have felt the same way—"I'm cutting carbs and avoiding sodas, but I'm not losing weight the way I would like to"—you now have the answer, or at least a big part of it. It's right under our collective nose. If we're avoiding Coke but biting into Colby, and cutting back on Dr Pepper but tucking into pepper jack, we're not going to succeed.

Sugar is just not the main issue. Although Americans trimmed their intake of sweeteners by 15 percent between 1999 and 2013, their cheese intake *rose* by about 16 percent during that same

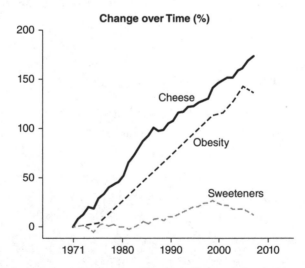

Source: U.S. Department of Agriculture, Economic Research Service, http://ers.usda.gov/data-products/food-availability-(per-capita)-data-system/.aspx#26705. Accessed November 14, 2015.

period. In fact, the amount of cheese on America's plate has been on a steady increase since World War II, and especially since the 1970s, when pizza and fast food arrived in a big way.

Have a look at the graph on page 32. You can see that obesity rates have almost exactly paralleled the increase in cheese consumption. The message is clear. Sugar is not exactly health food, but it is not the principal cause of weight problems. If we ignore the contribution of other food products—especially cheese— we are dooming ourselves to failure.

The Fat Lobby Fights Back

The producers of fatty foods have fought back. Yes, there's a lot of fat in cheese, they will agree. That's undeniable. But fat doesn't make you fat, they will assert. For years, Robert Atkins promoted a diet that included fatty meats and cream, but omitted starchy and sugary foods on the theory that less carbohydrate would mean weight loss. In practice, that meant that if you leave out fruit, bread, pasta, rice, potatoes, beans, cookies, cakes, and every other carbohydrate food, you'll lose weight. But it turned out that it worked only if dieters cut out so many foods that their total calories fell. Atkins sold millions of books but left many disappointed readers in his wake.

Because the Atkins low-carb diet relied on meat, eggs, and other fatty, cholesterol-laden foods, it was a recipe for heart problems. Normally, weight loss is supposed to bring cholesterol levels down. But clinical studies showed that, for about one in three Atkins dieters, cholesterol levels rose, sometimes to a frightening degree.

The low-carb camp never had an especially good answer for the fact that people in Japan and China, whose traditional diets included plenty of high-carbohydrate rice and noodles, were slim and healthy. And it was not just people laboring in the fields who stayed slim. Accountants, barbers, librarians, and bus drivers were thin, too, even though they were not working up a sweat. The fact is, rice just does not make you fat.

That all changed when American fast-food chains invaded these countries. As meat and cheese pushed rice off the table, waistlines quickly expanded, and diabetes and other health problems became epidemics. Fatty foods are loaded with calories, and cheese is about as fatty and calorie-packed as they come.

Let's Really Put It to the Test

So, does cutting out cheese and other fatty foods help? In 2012, a group of British researchers decided to look at *every* research study ever done in which researchers asked participants to cut down on fatty foods.[11] And they zeroed in specifically on studies where the goal was not to try to lose weight. People might have cut back on fatty foods to protect their hearts or prevent cancer, for example. It turned out that there were 33 studies published between 1960 and 2009, including 73,589 participants. In almost every study, people who cut down on fatty foods lost weight, even if they were not trying to cut calories. And the more they cut out fatty foods, the more weight they lost—a person who made a modest effort at cutting back on fat lost a modest amount of weight. Those who cut out more fatty foods lost more weight.

Three years later, the research team took a fresh look at the new studies that examined the issue. And the result was the same: Cutting out fatty foods leads to weight loss, and the more you cut, the more you lose.[12] Participants lost weight and their waistlines shrank in nearly every study.

For anyone who remains skeptical, researchers at the National

Institutes of Health examined the fat-versus-carbohydrate question especially rigorously. They asked nineteen overweight volunteers to move into the NIH Metabolic Clinical Research Unit for a tightly controlled experiment.[13] All of their meals were carefully prepared, and everything they ate was monitored and recorded. For six days, the volunteers had a reduced-calorie *low-fat* diet. And for a separate six-day period, they had a reduced-calorie *low-carbohydrate* diet. Both diets had exactly the same number of calories, but one was low-fat and the other was low-carb.

So, what happened? The low-fat diet led to significantly more fat loss, compared with the low-carbohydrate diet. The low-fat phase trimmed just over a pound of body fat in six days, compared with about half that amount on the low-carbohydrate diet. Six days is not long, and a pound of fat loss is not huge. But at that pace, you can imagine what would happen over a year's time.

Trimming Down, Feeling Great

If you are looking for power to trim away fat, now you have it. Instead of eating a food that nature made to fatten a calf, you can de-cheese your menu and de-fat your waistline.

So why doesn't everyone throw out the cheese and slim down? Back in Philadelphia, Geno reflects on what a cheeseless diet would mean. "I would feel deprived," he said. And it's true. It would rule out cheese fries, mac and cheese, and chicken cutlets breaded with cheese and then fried.

But keeping these foods means paying a serious price. Geno has had two surgeries, first a lap band, then a sleeve gastrectomy, with the result that he can eat only a tiny amount at a time. He also works out five days a week, aiming to burn away those extra calories. And he is not yet where he wants to be. "Unfortunately, I'm at a plateau. I'm still fighting it every day," he said.

Saying good-bye to cheese does mean leaving some old favorites behind. But new tastes quickly take their place. And it is also phenomenally easy—no surgery, no tiny portions, and not even any exercise, unless you feel like it.

So why doesn't everyone toss out the cheese? It's almost like there is something addictive in it. In the next chapter, we will see what that is. We will look at what it is about cheese that can get you hooked—and how to get back in charge.

CHAPTER 3

How Cheese Keeps You Hooked

Which foods do you find most addictive? That's the question University of Michigan researchers asked. The idea was, which foods lead you to lose control over how much you eat? Which ones are hard to limit? Which ones do you eat despite negative consequences? The researchers surveyed 384 people,[1] and here is what they found:

Problem food #5 is ice cream.

Problem food #4 is cookies.

Chips and chocolate were tied for #3 and #2.

But the most problematic food of all was—drumroll, please—pizza. Yes, gooey cheese melting over a hot crust and dribbling down your fingers—it beat everything else.

And here is what matters: The question was not, which foods do you especially *like*, or which foods leave you feeling good and satisfied. Rather, the question was, which foods do you have a problem with? Which ones lead you into overeating, gaining weight, and feeling lousy? Which foods seduce you, then leave you with regrets?

So, why did pizza top the list? Why are we so often tempted to dig in and overdo it?

Three reasons: salt, grease, and opiates.

As you have no doubt experienced, salty foods can be habit-forming. French fries, salted peanuts, pretzels, and other salty foods are hard to resist, and food manufacturers know that adding salt to a recipe adds cash to the register. A Lay's potato chips commercial in the 1960s said, "Bet you can't eat one"— meaning it's impossible to eat *just* one. Once the first salty chip passes your lips, you want more and more.

Your body does need some salt—about a gram and a half per day, according to U.S. health guidelines. In prehistoric times, however, salt was not so easy to come by. After all, potato chips and pretzels had not yet been invented. So people who managed to get their hands on salt were more likely to survive. Your neurological circuitry is set up to detect it, crave it, and jump in when you've found it.

As you will remember from fifth-grade biology, your tongue is very sensitive to the taste of salt. And brain scanning studies show that your brain is extra attuned to it, too.[2] Deep inside the brain, in what is commonly called the "reward center," brain cells make the feel-good neurotransmitter *dopamine*, and in certain situations it floods out of the cells, stimulating neighboring cells. If you find a particularly abundant source of food, your brain rewards you by releasing some dopamine. If you were to have—shall we say—a romantic, intimate encounter, your brain would have a similar reaction. It would give you more dopamine. Dopamine rewards you for doing things that help you or your progeny to live on. And scientists believe that dopamine plays a role in our desire for salt.[3]

So is there really a lot of salt in pizza? A fourteen-inch Domino's cheese pizza has—catch this—*3,391 milligrams of sodium.*[4] Just one slice delivers 400 milligrams. It's in the crust and in the toppings, and there is a lot in the cheese. So salt is one of the reasons that pizza attracts us.

Pizza is also greasy, and that greasy-salty combination seems to get us hooked, too, just as it does for chips, fries, and onion rings. But pizza has one more thing. It has cheese, and cheese not only contributes its own load of salt and grease. It also contains traces of a very special kind of opiate.

Casomorphins

In Chapter 1, I briefly mentioned *casein*, the protein that is concentrated in cheese. And casein has some secrets to tell.

If you were to look at a protein molecule with a powerful microscope, it would look like a long string of beads. Each "bead" is a protein building block called an *amino acid*, and, during digestion, the individual amino acids come apart and are absorbed into your bloodstream so that your body can use them to build proteins of its own.

So the calf digests the proteins in milk, breaking apart the chain of beads and using these amino acids to build skin cells, muscle cells, organs, and the other parts of the body.

However, casein is an unusual protein. While it does break apart to release individual beads, it also releases longer fragments—chains that might be four, five, or seven amino acid beads in length. These casein fragments are called *casomorphins*—that is, casein-derived morphine-like compounds.

And they can attach to the same brain receptors that heroin and other narcotics attach to.

In other words, dairy protein has opiate molecules built right into it.

Opiates in dairy products? What the heck are they doing there? you might ask. Well, imagine if a calf did not want to nurse. Or if a human baby was not interested in nursing. They would not do very well. So, along with protein, fat, sugar, and a sprinkling of hormones, milk contains opiates that reward the baby for nursing.

Have you ever looked at a nursing baby's face? The infant has a look of great intensity and then collapses into sleep. Of course, we imagine that to be the beauty of the mother-infant bond. But the fact is, mother's milk delivers a mild drug to the child, albeit in a benign and loving way. If that sounds coldly biological, it pays to remember that nature never leaves anything as important as a baby's survival to chance.

Opiates have a calming effect, and they also cause the brain to release dopamine, leading to a sense of reward and pleasure.

A cup of milk contains about 7.7 grams of protein, 80 percent of which is casein, more or less. Turning it into Cheddar cheese multiplies the protein content seven-fold, to 56 grams. It is the

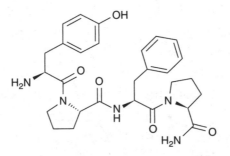

Morphiceptin, a casomorphin with the
formula Tyr-Pro-Phe-Pro.

most concentrated form of casein in any food in the grocery store.

Call it dairy crack. Just as cocaine manufacturers have found ways to turn an addictive drug (cocaine) into an extremely addictive one (crack), dairy producers have found their own ways to keep you coming back. In the Middle Ages, cheese makers had no idea that cheese might concentrate milk's addictive qualities. But today's cheese industry knows all about cheese craving and is eager to exploit it, as we will see in Chapter 8. It is doing its level best to trigger cheese craving in vulnerable people.

Sniffing Out Cheese

At a cost of £1.25 million, England's Manchester Airport built a facility to house drug-sniffing dogs, and in 2016, the independent chief inspector of borders and immigration reported on how the new drug detection program was working. It turned out that the dogs were not especially interested in finding heroin or cocaine. During the entire inspection period, they did not pick out either one. What did they go for? Cheese—and sausage. They found lots of both in the luggage of returning British holidaymakers.[5]

Why People Wax On about Love, Wine, and Roquefort

One peculiarity about dopamine: It makes you feel attracted to whatever elicited it. To see what I mean, do you remember your first sip of beer or first puff on a cigarette? Chances are they were not especially pleasant. But beer's bitter taste is quickly followed by alcohol working its mischief on your brain. As alcohol triggers the release of dopamine, dopamine makes you appreciate and like it. Soon, that bitter beer taste becomes attractive and, on a hot summer day, there is nothing a beer drinker wants more than a tall cold one.

Ditto for cigarettes. The first time anyone tries a cigarette, that puff is pretty harsh. But as nicotine enters the brain, it triggers dopamine release, too, and soon the smell and taste of cigarettes become attractive, even insistent.

So as casomorphins reach the brain of a nursing baby and trigger dopamine release, the baby attaches more and more to Mom. And if the casomorphins came, not from Mom, but from a slice of cheese, it would become attractive, too.

One more thing: Dopamine sometimes makes us confuse addiction with friendship. In the same way that alcoholics describe the bottle as their friend, and chocolate lovers sometimes turn to chocolate when they are lonely, as if chocolate can make up for a lack of human contact. That's dopamine at work. Dopamine can also turn the unwashed-feet smell of strong cheese from repulsive to attractive and convince us that, even if our human friends let us down, this gloppy load of calories still cares about us.

Paying a Price

I have heard from many, many people who feel hooked on cheese. Some have been participants in our research studies. As we help them to change their diets to tackle weight problems, diabetes, high cholesterol, or high blood pressure, many report that getting away from cheese is harder than breaking away from other foods.

You might have found the same thing. Let me share with you the experiences some folks have described to me. See if they sound familiar.

Cheri

Cheri is a software engineer. She is married and has three grown children. And she put it bluntly: "I can't seem to leave the cheese alone."

"When I was little, we didn't eat cheese," she said. "We didn't have fast food or pizza or cheese all over everything like it is today. But when I was thirteen or fourteen, we started having grilled cheese sandwiches and macaroni and cheese with Velveeta. And I loved it."

Cheese started to figure big on the family table. As long as she was physically active, her weight stayed in bounds. But in her mid-twenties, things started to change. She was raising her children and not exercising, and her eating habits began to take a toll. "I started putting on about 10 pounds a year, and eventually I hit 319 pounds." On a five-foot, five-inch frame, that meant a body mass index of 53, well into the obese range.

"I tried every diet on the planet, plus exercising. And I'd lose 10 or 20 pounds and then gain it all back, over and over."

Cheese called her name, and still does. "I love feta on a salad, Mexican-style shredded cheese in tacos, enchiladas, or quesadillas, or on baked potatoes. I love pepper jack on a sandwich or with crackers, or just by itself."

One day, she reported some peculiar feelings in her chest to her doctor, who promptly ordered an EKG and an angiogram—a special X-ray of the heart. She had significantly narrowed coronary arteries. So she went into the hospital and came out with a stent in a coronary artery, along with medications for high cholesterol, high blood pressure, and diabetes—a disease she had not known she had. "It was a rough week," she said. Her doctor also encouraged her to stop yo-yo dieting, saying that recurrent weight changes could damage her heart.

"I realized that I was on same path as my dad. He had had a heart attack at age forty-nine and another one at fifty-five. And at sixty, he had a major stroke that left him paralyzed on his right side and unable to speak. He lived that way for another twenty-two years."

One day, Cheri saw a notice at work for a vegan nutrition and cooking class. She had heard that a vegan diet could reverse heart disease, so she jumped at the chance. And she loved it. Tossing out meat and eggs, she lost 35 pounds over the next year. Her cholesterol fell, her doctor stopped her cholesterol medications, and she felt great.

But one thing was holding her back. "I can't get away from cheese. It is like a compulsion. Sometimes I go for weeks without it, but then I just have to have it. I can't figure it out."

The cravings hit especially strongly at night. "If I'm home alone, I get bored and maybe lonely. And I put some cheese on popcorn or on a tortilla, or have just plain shredded cheese." There is plenty of cheese in the refrigerator to tempt her, left by her husband who did not join her in the vegan class. He is overweight, too, and has diabetes and high cholesterol.

"When I have it, I feel much better, but then I feel guilty. It feels like an addiction. It's like there is something in it that my body is craving."

Ron

Ron is a real estate agent. When he was growing up in Houston and Phoenix, his diet was, in a word, awful. There was lots of junk food at home, and cheese was a big part of it—nothing fancy, just lots of grilled cheese sandwiches, eggs and cheese, pizza, and similar fare.

As a youngster, Ron was athletic, playing baseball and running track, and he was in good shape, except for one thing. He had severe sinus allergies. "I had excruciating sinus headaches, my nose was running constantly, I had trouble concentrating in school, and I was falling asleep." He also had frequent colds and flus. "I took over-the-counter allergy medications and, in my toddler and pre-teen years, I always seemed to need penicillin. I thought the problem must be environmental and never figured that it was related to my diet."

Ron's love for cheese continued in adulthood, with Cheddar, provolone, Brie, Swiss, and aged cheese of any kind. "I loved provolone on tuna sandwiches, Swiss on turkey sandwiches, pizza with extra cheese, cottage cheese, American cheese sandwiches with mayonnaise, cheeseburgers, mac and cheese, potatoes au gratin, eggplant and chicken parmigiana—you get the idea. It just tasted great and had great texture."

But one day, he picked up a book that advocated getting away from meat and dairy products. And he began putting two and two together. As he experimented with some diet improvements, two things came into focus. First, the connection with his health became clear. When he avoided dairy products—especially cheese—his sinus problems and allergies disappeared, and he also started contemplating what all the fat, cholesterol, and salt in the cheese had been doing to his arteries. Second, he found that avoiding cheese was *hard*. "If I saw it or smelled it, it was like, oh my God, I've got to get some. It's like nicotine or anything else that's addictive. It was the hardest thing to even think about getting rid of it."

If he was at a party where cheese was served, he had to avoid going near it. There were times when he gave in, and he came to realize that, for him, cheese was, for all intents and purposes, an addiction. It was all the harder that his wife was dealing with much the same issue. She had managed to shift to almond milk and soy yogurt, but felt addicted to cheese. She simply could not imagine avoiding it.

As time has gone on, though, keeping Ron's resolve has gotten easier. He has become more and more motivated to take care of his own health, and he has also learned of the unsavory ways the dairy industry treats animals. (More on that in Chapter 7.) "Now when I see people eating it, instead of being attracted to it, I'm concerned about what they are doing to themselves. I want to say, 'Let's talk.'

"When I was eating cheese and other junk foods, I felt lethargic, I had constant sinus problems, and I realized it was related to what I was eating. Breaking the habit was hard, but it has made an enormous difference."

Alan

Alan grew up in the San Francisco Bay Area in a Chinese family. Home dinners were traditional rice-based Chinese dishes. But lunches were Westernized fare, often including pizza, and the family refrigerator was stocked with American slices or supermarket Cheddar. During a junior high school trip to France and Switzerland, and later during a year-long stay in Germany as an exchange student, he learned about cheeses he had not seen back home. Later on, in graduate school, he and his wife explored many new foods, and his fondness for cheese grew.

"I like a really ripe Brie or stinky Camembert, a strong Emmentaler or Gruyère, a nice Manchego, petit Basque, aged Gouda, or anything blue. It seems that it's the salty, fermented taste and the feel of it that I like."

Unfortunately, he paid a price. "I have high cholesterol," he said. "I take medication for it, and even then, it is barely into the normal range. I also have high blood pressure, and I take medication for that, too." Cheese is a classic contributor to both problems, with its load of saturated fat, cholesterol, and sodium, as we will see in Chapter 5.

So what about the idea of not eating it? "Oh, no. I enjoy it too much. Am I addicted? I don't know, but life without cheese would be a dreary place."

Cheese, Bacon, Cheese, and Bacon—on a Burger

In 2015, the Wendy's fast-food chain unveiled a new combo meal with cheese cravers in mind. For just under seven dollars, you could bring home a burger topped with Gouda cheese, Gruyère cheese sauce, three strips of bacon, onions, lettuce, tomato, and garlic aioli, along with French fries coated with Gruyère and sprinkled with bacon bits.

Casomorphins and the Brain

Are casomorphins for real? Yes, they are. But some researchers have legitimately asked whether they can really affect the brain. First of all, to get to the brain, they first need to get into the bloodstream. Could molecules as big as casomorphins do that?

It's a valid question. However, a disturbing answer came from the cries of human babies. Many breast-feeding mothers recognize that what they eat can make their babies colicky, and among the most common culprits is cow's milk. When Mom drinks cow's milk, her breast-feeding baby can sometimes get a painfully upset stomach.[6] What that means is the food molecules are passing from the mother's digestive tract, into her bloodstream, and eventually into her milk.

Researchers from Washington University in St. Louis confirmed that, yes, even very large protein molecules in cow's milk can pass from a mother's digestive tract, into her bloodstream, and then into her own breast tissue, ending up in her own milk in quantities that are large enough to cause painful colic in her baby.[7]

To see if this applies to casomorphins, researchers conducted test-tube studies with intestinal cells and found that, indeed, casomorphins can pass through.[8] In 2009, researchers found human casomorphins in the bloodstreams of breast-fed infants and bovine casomorphins in the bloodstreams of bottle-fed babies.[9] They were looking for them because of the possibility that bovine casomorphins might play a role in brain disorders, such as autism. That's another story. But these findings suggest that, yes, milk proteins—including casomorphins—can indeed pass from the digestive tract into the bloodstream, at least under certain circumstances.

But can they get to the brain? I recently attended a health conference at which a reporter angrily dismissed the notion of cheese addiction. She pointed out that the *blood-brain barrier* stops things like dairy opiates from entering the brain. And indeed, the tiny blood vessels coursing through the brain do not permit just anything and everything to pass into the brain. The cells that make up the delicate vessel walls are like border guards, doing their best to regulate what gets through.

However, in 2009, the European Food Safety Authority addressed this very question. Can opiates from milk pass into the bloodstream and, from there, into the brain? And while they concluded that the research picture was far from perfect, yes, milk-derived opiates can pass from the digestive tract into the blood, and that it is indeed possible that they may cross into the brain.[10]

The passage of milk proteins into the brain has been studied in another way—one you would never have predicted: in women suffering with psychiatric problems after childbirth.

Breast Milk and Postpartum Psychosis

Many women have mood changes after giving birth—not surprising, given the hormone changes, sleeplessness, and pain they have been through. But about one in a thousand has a much more severe reaction called *postpartum psychosis*. It starts in the days or weeks after delivery and manifests as insomnia, restlessness, irritability, and depression, and can rapidly shift into delusions and hallucinations.

In 1984, Swedish researchers analyzed cerebrospinal fluid samples from eleven women with postpartum psychosis. Cerebrospinal fluid is the clear, watery substance that bathes the central nervous system, all the way from the brain to the bottom of the spinal cord. The women ranged in age from twenty-one to thirty-six, and all were lactating. Samples from four of the eleven had high levels of opiates that turned out to be casomorphins.[11]

Where had the casomorphins come from? The researchers checked blood samples. The analyses showed that, yes, casomorphins were there, too. So apparently, they passed from the bloodstream into the cerebrospinal fluid and brain.

But how did they get into the blood?

Here is what was apparently happening: The women were, of course, producing breast milk. And inside their breasts, casein molecules had broken apart, producing casomorphins that then passed from their breast tissue into their bloodstreams. Eventually, they found their way into the mothers' cerebrospinal fluid. And the theory is that it triggered their psychotic symptoms.

Checking samples from a larger group of lactating women, the researchers found that casomorphins turn up routinely in their blood and cerebrospinal fluid. So, when it comes to these opiates, the blood-brain barrier is barely a barrier at all. Casomorphins pass readily from the blood into the brain.[12]

It is peculiar to imagine that a woman's breast tissue could release enough casomorphins into the bloodstream to affect the brain, but that sequence of events apparently does occur. Rather than being an accident, the passage of casomorphins from the breast into the brain may actually have some biological benefits, providing a calming effect for both mother and infant. And the Swedish researchers speculate that they may help the mother focus her attention on the baby.

Postpartum psychosis may represent a toxic effect when the amount of casomorphins in the bloodstream is too high, or perhaps the effect of opiates in individuals predisposed to psychosis.

Hooked on Cheese

Most people are not lactating, needless to say. So there is no breast-tissue factory releasing casein into their blood. But a great many are eating cheese, and lots of it, on a daily basis. In all probability, traces of casomorphins are passing into their blood and into their brains.

This does not mean that cheese will render you psychotic; it may be that other genetic predispositions are necessary for that reaction to occur. But what is not at all unlikely is that cheese will get its clutches on your brain just enough to make you want more. And when you have a choice of adding cheese to a sandwich, salad, or pizza, as opposed to leaving it off, your cheese-addicted brain will call out as insistently as a baby wailing for the breast.

So, Am I a Cheese Addict?

Okay, so you crave cheese, and now you know that it's not just tasty; it actually contains concentrated opiates, along with salt and grease, that tend to keep us hooked. Does that mean you're addicted?

Well, that's a strong word. Let's see how the American Psychiatric Association defines these sorts of things. In its *Diagnostic and Statistical Manual of Mental Disorders, 5th Edition*, the APA lists a broad range of substance-use disorders, including problems with opiates, alcohol, caffeine, tobacco, other recreational drugs, and gambling.[13] For a diagnosis of Opioid Use Disorder, you need to meet at least two criteria from a list that includes the following signs, among others:

- Taking in larger amounts than intended.
- Persistent desire or unsuccessful attempts to cut down or control use.
- Craving or strong desire for the substance.
- Continued use despite having a problem that has been caused or exacerbated by the substance.

There are more serious signs, too, for more severe cases, such as being unable to carry out work obligations due to substance use or withdrawal symptoms. I hope these do not apply to you. But the more mundane aspects—taking in larger amounts than intended, persistent desire, unsuccessful efforts to cut down, cravings, and continuing to use it despite negative consequences—do these sound familiar? They sound a bit like the pizza craving we discussed at the beginning of this chapter, don't they?

Many people feel they are addicted to foods—chocolate,

sugar, or just eating in general—and some psychiatrists have written about the phenomenon.[14] Although some health professionals are reluctant to suggest that being hooked on foods is similar to being hooked on drugs, many people who have food-related problems say that it really does feel very much like any other addiction. Some go further, saying that ignoring the addictive characteristics of certain foods makes it that much harder to tackle the problem.

My sense is that it helps to set aside moralistic tones and an overly dogmatic stance. Instead, let's ask ourselves: Am I hooked on something that is hurting me? If that is your situation, that's all you need to know. And if you'd like to differentiate between *liking* something and *being hooked* on it, try these three questions:

1. Do you have it every day, and especially at about the same time of day?
2. Do you crave it and/or miss it when it's gone?
3. Are you paying a price for it, especially with regard to your health?

As these questions suggest, addictions tend to be on cycles. We fall into patterns that recur day after day. They involve craving—an intense desire for something, or intensely missing it when it's gone. Finally, they hurt us. Some things hurt us a little—caffeine's withdrawal effects, for example. Others hurt us a lot—drugs, alcohol, and cigarettes can be in that category. Food problems can range from minor to major, and sometimes they are life-threatening. Whether you're hooked and how much harm it may be causing—that's for you to decide.

Why does it matter? Because if you feel like you're hooked, you can take advantage of what we know about breaking other habits. Just as smokers quickly learn that it is much easier to simply avoid cigarettes than to try to have them "in moderation," you will likely find that the same is true of foods that call your name. You may also find that social support is especially helpful and that avoiding trigger situations is, too.

The good news is that it is easy to find delightful substitutes for unhealthful foods. Have a look at Chapter 10 and the recipe section.

CHAPTER 4

Hidden Hormone Effects

When Katherine finished her tour of duty in Iraq, she was slim and reasonably healthy. Let's face it: It is not easy to gain weight when you're working hard in 120°F heat. As an Air Force aerospace engineer, Katherine designed missiles and military bases and had been among the first to go into Iraq in 2003.

Coming home meant returning to the foods of her Louisiana childhood: gumbo, shrimp, and cheesy casseroles. Cheese had a special place in her life. She fell into the odd habit of having a double cheeseburger for breakfast and snacked on *Cheetos* later in the day. And she especially loved macaroni and cheese, made with extra butter. For Christmas, a friend gave her an entire case of Kraft macaroni and cheese dinners—forty-eight boxes—and she ate a box a day for forty-eight days. At Mexican restaurants, she dug into hot melted *queso* flavored with bits of meat and peppers. Nachos and quesadillas, too.

In truth, her diet was not so different from those of other

people she knew, and her portions were not out of bounds. But like many of her friends, she found herself gaining weight over time. She also started to experience pain in her abdomen. It waxed and waned with her menstrual cycle, and it gradually worsened. Eventually, her gynecologist scheduled her for a laparoscopy, a technique for looking into the abdomen through a small incision. And that made the diagnosis. Katherine had endometriosis—collections of cells from the uterus that ended up planting in various places in her abdomen, attaching to her ovaries and even her intestinal tract. As women with endometriosis will tell you, the pain can sometimes be excruciating. It can be hard to just get out of bed, let alone go to work or go out with friends. It can also lead to infertility.

Katherine was miserable, and things were not getting better. Her doctor concluded that the only solution was a hysterectomy.

Okay. She had wanted to have children, but if a hysterectomy was the only treatment for her illness, she resolved herself to it. She proceeded with plans for the operation.

But then a friend suggested something completely different. After all, foods are known to affect hormones in various ways. Why not try a diet change?

Halfheartedly, but with no other option, she sought out the advice of a nutrition counselor, who encouraged her to set aside dairy products, meat, and eggs, and try a vegan diet. He also suggested a number of traditional Asian foods—miso soup, brown rice, broccoli, and adzuki beans.

During the diet experiment, she missed her favorite foods, especially cheese and everything she had made with it. But very soon she felt remarkably better. Not only did pounds start melting away; her symptoms faded, too. Something was definitely happening. After six weeks, she went back to her doctor for a repeat laparoscopy. Her doctor was stunned. Her disease had regressed dramatically, so much so that she did not need a hysterectomy after all.

When the doctor told Katherine the news, she broke into tears. She had hoped that there was some explanation for her improvement other than the diet changes she had made—some explanation that could mean she would not have to say a permanent good-bye to her favorite, albeit unhealthful, foods. But she now realized that cheese and junk food were the *cause* of her problem. These foods meant pain and infertility. "I was either going to have cheese or have kids—that was the choice. I realized that I did this to myself, and now I had to decide what I was going to do about it."

In the waiting room, the doctor shared the good news with her husband, too. The endometriosis was all but gone. And her husband said, yes, he had been amazed to see how quickly the diet change had worked.

No way, the doctor said. It could not have been her new diet; that's just not possible. Foods don't cause endometriosis, and a diet change could never have led to this great an improvement. Really? Then, what could have made the difference, her husband asked. There was only one explanation, the doctor said: It must have been a miracle. "Miracles happen all the time," he explained.

Miracle or not, Katherine stuck with her new way of eating. Her weight continued to improve—down 55 pounds in six months. Her cholesterol dropped 80 points. Painful breast cysts went away. And as her symptoms melted away, she felt better emotionally, too. No more mood roller coasters.

Once in a while, she deviated from her resolve, adding a slice of cheese to a veggie burger or digging into other cheesy foods.

And these dietary indiscretions caused her pain and breast tenderness to quickly return and made her cycle noticeably heavier. She discovered that acne, which had bothered her for years but went away on her healthy diet, promptly returned if she flirted with cheese. "It was as if my body was trying to reject the dairy and get it out of my body."

She resolved to stick to her new way of eating, and soon she came to love the new foods and tastes she was discovering. About that surgery? She never had it. She did not need it.

Katherine and her husband now have two children, aged three and five. Yes, she serves them macaroni and other childhood favorites, but these foods are prepared differently. There's not a speck of cheese on anything. She educates her children on the dangers of cheese and fills their lunchboxes with healthier alternatives. She gets the taste of cheese from nutritional yeast and other ingredients, and has found many other ways to combine the best of health with the best of taste. You'll learn how to do the same in the recipe section of this book.

Understanding Hormones

A hormone is a natural chemical made in the body that controls the function of cells and organs. Insulin, for example, is made in your pancreas. It travels to your muscles and liver to control your blood sugar. Similarly, the adrenal glands sitting on top of your kidneys make epinephrine (also called adrenaline) to speed up your heart, widen your pupils, raise your blood sugar, and get you ready to flee from danger or to fight, as the case may be. Hormones are chemical messengers that tell the cells and organs what to do.

The estrogens—female sex hormones—produced in a woman's body are responsible for breast development and many of the changes that occur in the monthly cycle. Small amounts of estrogens in the bloodstream are normal, of course. But, as we will see, food choices can influence the amount of estrogens in your body, and too much estrogen in the bloodstream can spell danger, as has been shown when hormones are used as medications. In a large government-funded health study, called the Women's Health Initiative, women who were given hormone "replacement" therapy were more likely to develop breast cancer compared with women not taking hormones (about 24 percent more).[1]

If you were to look up the risks of Premarin—a common hormone preparation prescribed for hot flashes and other menopausal symptoms—on the manufacturer's website, you would find a long list of warnings about breast cancer, uterine cancer, strokes, blood clots, heart attacks, and dementia.[2] Premarin is made from the urine of pregnant horses (its name is short for "pregnant mare's urine"), rather than cows, but it is safe to assume that estrogens from pregnant cows carry similar risks, depending on the dose. More on that below.

Some of these risks have been known for decades. Starting in 1956, estrogens were used to slow the growth of adolescent girls who appeared to be growing too quickly. The idea was that a girl might grow "too tall to attract a husband or work as a flight attendant." Injections of high-dose estrogens halted their growth, but caused serious side effects: early puberty, weight gain, infertility, blood clots, liver problems, and hormone-related cancers.

Female hormones can work mischief in a man's body, too. In the same way that estrogens cause fat to deposit in the breasts of an adolescent girl, the same process can begin in a man who has too much estrogen in his blood, as you will see on just about any beach in America.

The bottom line is that nature builds hormones into our bodies in tiny amounts for specific functions. Small increases can cause serious problems, and big increases can spell disaster.

Hormones in Dairy Products

Dairy products affect hormone functions in many ways, directly and indirectly. Let's start with estrogens themselves. Estrogens are in milk when it comes from the cow and when you pour it on your cereal. They won't show up in milk advertisements or appear on the package label, because the Food and Drug Administration does not require dairies to report them. Here is where they come from:

To point out the obvious, most cows do not produce milk, any more than most women do. They make milk only if they have been pregnant. So farmers impregnate their cows every year. Surprising as it sounds, much of the milk that goes into the dairy products you buy—perhaps most of it—comes from pregnant cows. So when you drink a glass of milk, have a bowl of ice cream, or chew a bit of cheese, you're getting traces of hormones that surge during pregnancy.

At Penn State University, researchers tested cow's milk samples for estrogens, including estrone, estrone sulfate, and estradiol.[3] Early in pregnancy, the hormone content of milk is low, but as the months go by, it quickly rises. The Penn State researchers found that, over the course of pregnancy, the amount of estradiol in milk jumped seventeen-fold, and estrone rose forty-five-fold. The difference is so big that a laboratory could easily tell you if a pail of milk came from a cow late in her pregnancy. Dairies and cheese makers do nothing to remove these hormones. They are passed along to you in milk and other dairy products.

Bovine Growth Hormone

You've probably heard that farmers sometimes inject bovine growth hormone into cattle to boost milk production. Also called *recombinant bovine somatotropin* (rBST), it is a genetically engineered product launched by Monsanto in 1994. The rationale for using it is that a cow's milk production peaks after about seventy days of lactation and then gradually declines, in part due to the fall of the number of milk-producing cells in her udder. Bovine growth hormone keeps more of these milk-producing cells functioning and directs nutrients toward milk production.

Growth hormone used illegally by athletes has side effects, and it has side effects for cows, too. In eight separate Monsanto studies, including 487 cows, growth hormone injections caused a 50 percent increase in mastitis—inflammation of the udder—typically leading to antibiotic treatment and various health complications for the cow. A post-approval monitoring program tracked twenty-eight herds, finding a 32 percent increase in mastitis among hormone-treated cows. The mastitis caused by the hormone injections is challenging to treat and results in much more antibiotic use, compared with typical mastitis cases that arise sporadically.[4]

As a result of these and other health concerns, bovine growth hormone is banned in Canada, the European Union, Australia, New Zealand, Japan, and Israel. But many U.S. dairy farms still use it.

Needless to say, many consumers are not so keen on drinking milk from cows injected with hormones, and some dairy companies have policies against the injections. However, some states have made it illegal for these producers to label milk as "hormone-free." Their rationale is that all milk has hormones. And that, of course, is true—if you drink milk or eat cheese, you are swallowing the cow's hormones. And, of course, if people knew the facts about hormone-treated cows, they might not buy the product.

Still, the amounts of female hormones in milk are small—far too small to affect our health, right? Well, that's not clear. Researchers in Melbourne, Australia, measured hormone levels in 766 postmenopausal women. Those whose diets included the most dairy products had 15 percent more estradiol circulating in their bloodstreams, compared with women consuming the least dairy products.[5]

Researchers at Kaiser Permanente in Oakland, California, examined the diets of 1,893 women participating in the Life After Cancer Epidemiology study, all of whom had been diagnosed with early-stage invasive breast cancer. Over the next twelve years, those who averaged just one-half to one serving of high-fat dairy products on a daily basis were 20 percent more likely to die of breast cancer, compared with those having little or no high-fat dairy products. And for women who consumed slightly more—at least a full serving of fatty dairy products on a daily basis—the risk of dying of breast cancer was 49 percent higher.[6]

Researchers at the University of Rochester looked at the effects on men. They tracked dairy intake in 189 male college students, and then checked sperm samples on each of them. It turned out that those eating the most dairy products, especially cheese and other fatty dairy products, were more likely to have abnormal sperm. Specifically, the morphology and motility—the shape and movement—of their sperm were abnormal. Fertility problems have been gradually increasing, the researchers noted.[7] Could the parallel rise in cheese consumption be part of the explanation?

The Rochester researchers then examined men attending a fertility clinic and zeroed in especially on cheese. The men who had the most cheese (ranging from one to two and a half servings per day) had a 28 percent lower sperm concentration, compared with men having less than about half a serving per day. They also had poorer sperm motility and morphology.[8]

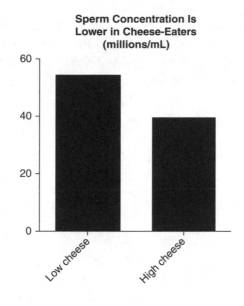

Sperm Concentration Is Lower in Cheese-Eaters (millions/mL)

Fat, Fiber, and Hormones

Dairy products contain hormones. But there are other ways that dairy products affect your hormone balance:

First, body fat builds hormones. Body fat is not an inert substance. It is living tissue, and one of the things it does is build estrogens. So if cheese makes you gain weight, that added body fat builds estrogens. In men, that can mean visible breast development, among other problems.

Second, fiber helps you eliminate hormones. Every minute of every day, your liver filters your blood, removing toxins and anything else that your body needs to get rid of. That includes excess hormones. The liver sends these unwanted compounds through a narrow tube called the bile duct into your intestinal tract. There, fiber (plant roughage) soaks them up and carries them out of the body with the wastes.

If your diet includes plenty of vegetables, fruits, beans, and whole grains, this system works fine. You'll have the fiber you

(continued)

need to rid yourself of excess hormones. But cheese is not a plant, so it has no fiber. Ditto for any other animal product. And that means that if your diet is filled with animal products, your body lacks the fiber you need to eliminate unwanted hormones.

Cancer researchers believe that this is part of why people whose diets are based on animal products tend to have higher rates of some cancers and why fiber reduces cancer risk. Fiber helps keep hormone levels in bounds.

Turning Health Around

Lest these problems seem simply theoretical, let me tell you about a woman who joined a research study that our team conducted. We were trying to see whether diet changes could reduce menstrual cramps. Many women get cramps each month, of course, and for most, they are manageable. For some, however, the pain can be so severe that it is hard to get through the day. We asked half the participants to follow a diet that was free of all animal products—no meat, no cheese or other dairy products, no eggs, and very little fat of any kind—for two months and then go back to their previous way of eating for two more months. The other half did the diets in the opposite order—their usual diets first, then the vegan diet.

The results came quickly. The women following their usual diets didn't get any benefits, needless to say. But when they adopted the plant-based diet, many found their pains diminishing or going away. In the group that had the plant-based diet first, many participants improved so much that they refused to go back to their previous way of eating when the study called for them to. They felt so good on their new way of eating, they did not want to go back to the foods that had hurt them for so many years.[9]

During the study, we wanted to make sure that our participants were not taking birth control pills, because the pill's hormonal effects would have confused the study results. So we asked them to use a different birth-control method—whatever method they chose. One participant said that she did not need birth control, because she was infertile. She and her husband had been trying for years to have a baby. They had been thoroughly evaluated and the problem was not her husband. She was infertile and had resigned herself to it.

As fate would have it, soon after she began the new diet she had something to tell me. "I have good news and bad news," she said. "The bad news is that I can't be in the study anymore. The good news is that I am pregnant." Needless to say, she and her husband were elated. She continued with the healthy diet, and several years later, she came to a lecture I was giving and introduced me to her three children.

So what made the difference? Was it because she dumped cheese from her diet? Yes, I believe that is part of the answer. And because her diet was so rich in healthful fiber, her hormones were likely able to get into better balance.

What about Soy?

Some people have ignored the hormones in cow's milk, and focused instead on the idea that there might be hormones in milk substitutes, especially soy milk. Here is what they are thinking:

Soybeans and many other foods contain natural compounds called *isoflavones*. Because their chemical structure vaguely resembles sex hormones, some have called these compounds *phytoestrogens*—meaning "plant estrogens" (*phyto* comes from the Greek word for "plant")—and have suggested that soy products might cause breast cancer, or make breast cancer progress.

(continued)

It turns out that the opposite is true. Rather than causing cancer, soy products appear to help prevent it. In 2008, researchers examined the relationship between soy products and breast cancer, combining the results of eight prior studies in a careful meta-analysis.[10] They looked especially at studies on Asians and Asian Americans, for whom soy milk and tofu would be familiar foods. It turned out that women consuming the most soy were 29 percent *less* likely to develop breast cancer, compared with women who neglected soy products. In 2014, a new meta-analysis was done, this one combining the results of 35 prior studies, and again, soy had a preventive effect, cutting breast cancer risk by 41 percent.[11]

Researchers have also studied what happens for women who had breast cancer already. Many women who have been treated for breast cancer are counseled by their well-meaning doctors to avoid soy products, on the theory that soybeans "have estrogens that can make cancer grow." Researchers have carefully examined this question. In 2012, the results from 9,514 breast cancer survivors were reported. And it turned out that, for those women consuming the most soy products, cancer was roughly 30 percent *less* likely to recur, compared with women who consumed little or no soy.[12] These studies show that, rather than encouraging cancer growth, soy milk, tofu, and other soy products actually help prevent cancer.

From my standpoint, soy products are not essential. But they are very handy for replacing milk, cheese, meat, and other products that carry serious health risks. And, if anything, soy products help prevent breast cancer and help women who have been treated for breast cancer to reduce the odds that cancer will come back.

Milk, Vitamin D, and Cancer

Dairy products have also been implicated in cancer for men. Prostate cancer is extremely common, so much so that, when I was in medical school I was taught that *all* men will get prostate cancer if they live long enough. That was an exaggeration, but you get the idea.

Studying a world map of prostate cancer, it soon becomes clear that the disease is actually rather rare in places like Japan, Thailand, and Hong Kong, where dairy products are not traditional foods (or at least it *was* rare before these countries began adopting Western eating habits). But it is common in countries where dairy products are routine parts of the diet—Switzerland, France, Norway, Sweden, Canada, and the U.S., among others.[13]

So Harvard researchers looked to see if the association holds up within the U.S. and whether men who do not yet have cancer are more likely to develop it if they consume dairy products. The Physicians' Health Study included 20,885 men, all of whom were cancer-free at the beginning of the study.[14] The researchers took detailed diet records and then followed the men over the next eleven years. And yes, those who had at least two and a half dairy servings per day had a 34 percent increased risk of developing prostate cancer.

A second Harvard study in a larger group—this one including 47,781 men—came to a similar conclusion.[15] In the Health Professionals Follow-Up Study, men who had more than two milk servings per day were 60 percent more likely to develop prostate cancer.

Why would dairy products be linked to cancer? Well, it pays to remember what milk is for. It helps a baby grow. It does that not only by supplying protein, sugar (lactose), and fat; it also stimulates the production of growth-promoting compounds in the baby's body.

Insulin-like growth factor, or IGF-I, is a substance in the bloodstream that promotes growth, as its name implies. Some IGF-I is produced within a baby's body naturally, and milk stimulates increased IGF-I production. Same for adults:

Milk-drinking boosts IGF-I levels in the blood. At Creighton University, researcher Robert Heaney asked a group of men and women, aged fifty-five to eighty-five, to drink three glasses of milk a day. Their IGF-I levels rose by about 10 percent, on average.[16] And that is worrisome, because test-tube studies show that IGF-I causes cancer cells to grow rapidly.

Back at Harvard, the researchers had taken blood samples from the Physicians' Health Study participants as the study was getting under way. And it turned out that the men who later developed cancer had more IGF-I in their blood when the study started ten years earlier.[17] The IGF-I difference between those with cancer and those who stayed cancer-free was about 10 percent—matching the difference in IGF-I levels between people who indulge in dairy products and those who do not. In other words, the evidence suggests that milk and other dairy products stimulate the production of IGF-I in the bloodstream and that, in turn, IGF-I promotes the growth of cancer cells.

Vitamin D and Cancer

Dairy products may increase cancer risk through a second mechanism, this one relating to vitamin D. Vitamin D is produced by sunlight on the skin. It is then activated in the liver and kidneys, and from there it circulates in the bloodstream.

Vitamin D's best-known job is to help the body absorb calcium. When you are low in calcium, your body activates more vitamin D to help your intestinal tract absorb more calcium from the foods you've eaten. When you have lots of calcium on board already, your body slows down its vitamin D activation, and so you absorb less calcium.

So far, so good. But vitamin D has another job, too, which is to protect you from cancer, scientists believe. And that's where dairy products work some mischief. If you are tucking into cheese, milk, and other dairy products, you're getting more calcium than your body needs. With all the calcium entering your bloodstream, *your body slows down its activation of vitamin D.* And with less vitamin D, your cancer risk increases. At least that is one of the key explanations for the link between dairy products and prostate cancer.

The role of foods in prostate cancer took on extra importance in a 2005 study conducted by Dr. Dean Ornish. Dr. Ornish had already shown that a plant-based diet, as part of a healthy lifestyle, could reverse heart disease, and he tested a similar regimen for men with prostate cancer.[18]

The men in the study had early-stage cancer, so they were able to defer treatment as long as their doctors tracked their cancer using a blood test called prostate-specific antigen, or PSA. If PSA levels stay fairly low, there is no need for surgery or other treatments. But if PSA rises sharply, cancer treatment (e.g., surgery to remove the prostate) may be needed.

Dr. Ornish invited ninety-three men to join the study. Half the men began a low-fat, vegan diet, along with moderate aerobic exercise and stress management, while the other half followed their usual diets. In the usual-diet group, PSA levels gradually worsened, which is typical in men with prostate cancer. For the average participant, PSA rose 6 percent in a year's time. But in the vegan group, PSA levels did not rise, on average. In fact, they fell 4 percent over a year's time. And although six men in the group that followed their usual diets had to leave the study to have their cancers treated, no one in the vegan group needed treatment during the study period.

Why did the diet change work? A low-fat, high-fiber, dairy-free diet is likely to help tame the hormones driving prostate cancer.

Fighting Back Against Cancer

The power of food can be far greater than you might have imagined. Let me share the experience of Ruth Heidrich. At age forty-seven, Ruth was living in Hawaii, working on a PhD in psychology. One day in the shower, she felt something no woman wants to find—a lump in her right breast.

She saw her physician, who quickly ordered a mammogram. To her relief, the scan showed no cancer. But just to be safe, the doctor recommended an annual mammogram. The following year, the test was again negative.

Unfortunately, in the third year, the mammogram showed the lump. It had slowly grown to the point where what had seemed innocuous was now showing its true colors. This was breast cancer, and it had been all along.

Ruth had surgery to remove the breast lump. But it turned out that the cancer had already spread to her bones, her left lung, and her liver. And there was no way to remove the deadly cancer that had spread throughout her body. Her doctor recommended chemotherapy and radiation. They were not cures, but they might help her buy a little time.

But then something remarkable happened. Ruth saw a newspaper notice about research on the role of diet in breast cancer. The researcher, Dr. John McDougall, explained that he was investigating whether a completely vegan diet—a diet with no animal products—could tackle breast cancer more effectively than chemotherapy or radiation. The idea was that foods affect hormone levels, sometimes in a harmful way, other times in a helpful way. By jettisoning the foods that tend to increase unhelpful hormones and favoring foods that help the body rid itself of hormones, perhaps cancer patients might benefit.

Ruth decided against chemotherapy and radiation and chose

a diet change instead. And it turned out to be easy: lots of vegetables, fruits, brown rice, whole-grain breads, oatmeal, and other healthful foods.

She also began a new program of exercise. She was already physically fit, but she pushed herself even more.

Within two months, the cancer began to disappear. Before long, her liver tests returned to normal. She never had chemotherapy or radiation. And her health rebounded.

Ruth became a strong advocate for health. Following a completely plant-based diet, she has run sixty-seven marathons and six Ironman Triathlons, and set several world age-group records. She wrote four books to let people know about her journey and about the power of foods for health. Now, more than three decades later, she is active and well, and remains a champion for a healthful diet.

Like Ruth, Katherine became eager to share what she had learned. She became a cooking instructor and began holding classes for women and men, many of whom have faced health problems that can be dramatically improved with a change in diet.

Health Surprises

It is safe to say that Katherine, Ruth, and many others like them were surprised to find that foods can have so much power. And the range of conditions linked to cheese in particular goes far beyond those we have touched on so far. Could your headaches, joint problems, or not-so-healthy-looking skin be caused by cheese? Let's take a look in the next chapter.

CHAPTER 5

Health Problems You Never Bargained For

We've seen how a daily dose of cheese can pack on the pounds and cause hormones to go haywire. But it can also lead to a surprising range of health problems, some subtle, others life-threatening. And in most cases you would never have guessed the cause. In this chapter, I will introduce you to Chad, Elizabeth, Lauren, Irene, Karen, Amy, and Ann—all real people whose lives were transformed once they learned the secrets you will find in this book. If you see yourself or someone you know in their stories, let me encourage you to use their experiences to revolutionize your own health.

Before we start, one note: You will notice that most of the health problems described in this chapter do not relate to fat or cholesterol, which are the usual issues with cheese and other dairy products. Those issues will be covered in the next chapter. The problems we will cover now relate to *protein*. Yes, dairy protein—which is concentrated in cheese—is a number-one suspect in a surprising range of sensitivities.

Eliminating Allergies and Asthma

Chad Sarno grew up near Portsmouth, New Hampshire, north of Boston and right on the water. Italian on his father's side and French Canadian on his mother's, he inherited a love of good food. His great-grandfather Rocco, arriving at Ellis Island, brought along a taste for ricotta-stuffed manicotti and many other family favorites.

As a youngster, Chad was big on sports—especially football—except that his games were often cut short. "I had terrible asthma," he said. "Allergies made me wheeze and cough, and that triggered the attacks." When asthma struck, it was terrifying. "It was like the vise on my father's work bench—a vise on my lungs. It was how I would imagine a heart attack to be."

Asthma is a serious disease. What Chad experienced as a vise around his lungs is actually hundreds of microscopic vises—muscles tightening on the airways all at the same time. Ten percent of Americans have asthma, and nine people die from it every day.

Chad took albuterol, prednisone, and theophylline. But his asthma was not going anywhere. Once, at a friend's home, dog dander triggered an asthma attack that was so severe the family had to call an ambulance. He was hospitalized at least a half-dozen times.

Sometimes asthma attacks just come out of the blue, and they can also be triggered by exercise. But often, the trigger is an allergy. An allergy is when your immune system is roused into action at the wrong time. Millions of white blood cells that are supposed to be attacking viruses and bacteria are now attacking you instead. They do this by sending out antibodies—protein "torpedoes" that cause all kinds of unpleasant reactions in your body: a rash, itching, sneezing, and asthma.

So how does all this relate to cheese? First of all, some people are allergic to milk and other dairy products, just as they can be allergic to eggs, peanuts, tree nuts, fish, wheat, or soy products, among other foods. But there is a second issue. Some people have observed that dairy products *seem to make other allergies worse*, and that avoiding dairy products seems to make other allergies improve or disappear. After getting away from milk products, some people notice that an allergy to animal dander, for example, diminishes or even goes away.

When Chad was around seventeen, he heard from a friend that dairy products can trigger breathing problems. In other words, the culprit might be his beloved manicotti and other dairy-based family favorites. And he started to connect the dots. He recalled, as a child, eating ice cream in the evening, and then coughing and wheezing at night. He decided to put the idea to the test. He cut out milk, cheese, and everything that had a trace of dairy in it. "It was not easy, but I wanted to try it," he said. "What choice did I have?"

The effect was dramatic. "Within a couple of months, my allergies went away and my wheezing just stopped." As time went on, he felt better and better. "Eventually, it was like I had never even had asthma. It was so liberating."

Chad encouraged his parents to try the same experiment. His mother stopped eating animal products altogether. Her cholesterol plummeted, and she began sharing plant-based recipes and cooking ideas with Chad since both have such a love for food.

Why Didn't Anyone Tell Me?

It took a long time for Chad to link dairy products to his asthma, and it's safe to say that most other people struggling with this disease have not heard about the link either. Why not?

Let's try a Google search using the term "asthma dairy." The search turns up, as item number one, a website from the National Asthma Council Australia, a "not-for-profit organization working to improve health outcomes and quality of life for people with asthma." Sounds great. And, as a matter of fact, it jumps right in with a section called "Dairy foods and asthma." Here is what it says:

> Dairy foods have often been suggested as a common trigger for asthma, but there is little scientific evidence to support this myth. A review summarizing the available evidence for the link between milk and asthma concluded: "current evidence does not directly link milk consumption and asthma." The National Asthma Council Australia also does not routinely recommend avoiding dairy foods as a way to manage asthma. They also advise that milk and dairy foods do not increase mucus.[1]

So this nonprofit discounts any link between dairy products and asthma. But it goes further:

> Unfortunately, most Australians are missing out on the health benefits that come from consuming milk, cheese and yogurt as they don't include enough dairy foods in their diet. It is estimated that eight out of 10 Australian adults and most Australian children need to increase their intake of the dairy food group in order to meet the Australian Dietary Guidelines.

Hmm. This is starting to smell funny. Let's click on the web page listing the council's corporate sponsors. There are eight: One is Dairy Australia. The others are drug companies—AstraZeneca, Boehringer Ingelheim, GlaxoSmithKline, Meda, Menarini, Mundipharma, and Novartis. In other words, the corporate sponsors of this website are organizations that make money if you continue to consume dairy products or continue to need medication.

There is a disturbing trend in the world of medicine in which food companies and drug manufacturers bankroll health organizations that dismiss—or sometimes actively oppose—approaches that can solve medical problems. You'll see this in diabetes, Alzheimer's disease, and many other conditions. With so much money clouding their vision, these organizations have lost sight of their purpose.

This is not to say that diet changes always solve the problem or that medications have no role. But if a simple change in diet can improve health or save a life, it is hard to justify keeping it hidden.

Okay, so what about that scientific evidence that the National Asthma Council Australia was talking about? Is the dairy-asthma link a myth or not? Let's have a look.

The scientific review that the council was referring to was published in *Canadian Family Physician* in 2012.[2] The review cited several studies, one of which took place in New York. Eleven adults with asthma drank either whole milk, skim milk, or water on separate days, and the researchers measured how well oxygen passed from their lungs into their bloodstream.[3] When the participants drank whole milk, their results deteriorated progressively over the three-hour test. The researchers concluded that, yes, something about milk fat is interfering with lung function in people with asthma.

The review also cited an English study including twenty-two children. Researchers carefully assessed the children's ability to breathe—measured as the *peak expiratory flow rate*, or PEFR. The test is simple. A child (or adult) blows through a tube, and it indicates how quickly he or she is exhaling. In asthma, breathing becomes labored, and the test shows how slow breathing has become. The children then began a milk- and egg-free diet. Eight weeks later, the test was repeated. The results were impressive: The children's lung function had improved by 22 percent, on average.[4] (Incidentally, the study coincided with Easter, so the researchers gave the kids chocolate bunnies from D&D Chocolates, a dairy-free chocolate company located in the aptly named town of Nuneaton.)

Neither of these studies was very large. But rather than discounting the role of dairy products in asthma, their results actually fit in with many people's experience, which is that getting away from dairy products can really help. By the way, a diet change does not work overnight. It takes time, and the reason is not hard to see: When allergens trigger the production of antibodies, it takes weeks for them to dissipate. This is important. Studies that eliminate dairy products for just a week or two or that test the effects of, say, a single glass of milk are likely to come up empty-handed.[5] Longer-term effects seem to be at work here.

A Lesson for Anyone Who Likes to Breathe

The apparent effect of dairy products on lung function holds a lesson for people who don't have asthma, but who want to be at their best. As we saw above, for the New York study volunteers, a glass of whole milk made it harder for oxygen to pass from their lungs into the bloodstreams. Other studies have shown that, once fat gets into your blood—whether it came from cheese or bacon or somewhere else—it makes it harder for oxygen to pass from your lungs into your bloodstream.[6] The effect is temporary and subtle, and most people would probably barely notice. But if endurance and energy matter to you, it is good to know that fatty foods seem to interfere with oxygenation.

The New York researchers speculated that there might be a particular problem with the fats in cow's milk. Dairy fat, they suggested, may increase the production of certain prostaglandins—compounds that play central roles in inflammation—in the lungs, interfering with oxygenation.[7]

So, Why Cheese?

Dairy products come in many forms, needless to say. But cheese is in a class by itself. As you know by now, the cheese-making process concentrates dairy fat and protein (as well as cholesterol, sodium, and calories). Here are the numbers: A cup of milk has 7.7 grams of protein, but a cup of melted Cheddar has 56. A cup of milk has 7.9 grams of fat; a cup of Cheddar has 81. So if dairy protein triggers allergies or makes other allergies worse, or if dairy fat impairs lung function, as the New York study suggested, cheese would be right at the top of the problem list.

Free of Asthma

Having seen the power of foods to cause and cure his asthma, Chad took a serious interest in nutrition and began to study culinary arts. He sought out ways to adapt his family favorites and discovered that it was possible to make "cheeses" from nuts and other simple ingredients. With cashews, bacterial cultures, and a little time, he found he could make a delicious cream cheese.

Eventually, Chad launched a restaurant, and then another and another—five in all, co-founded a website dedicated to healthful eating, called Wicked Healthy, with his brother Derek, built a plant-based professional certification cooking course for Rouxbe, the online culinary school, and helped launch a cooking instruction program for doctors to share with patients, called Culinary Rx (https://plantrician.rouxbe.com).

Today, Chad and his wife live with his ten-year-old daughter, a new baby boy, a boxer named Rocky, and a cat named Milo. "I have no allergies anymore at all. Not to animals, not to seasons, or anything else."

Other Respiratory Problems

Some 3,500 miles away, Elizabeth had much the same problem. Growing up in England, Elizabeth read storybooks about Heidi, the Swiss orphan girl who milked goats and ate cheese with bread straight from the oven. "As a little girl, I thought it would be fabulous to skip about in the mountains and to eat like that."

Elizabeth started her day with a half-inch of condensed milk ("condenny") in a teacup that she drowned with scalding hot tea. Later on, her father taught her to love cheese. No Velveeta for them. It was Wensleydale, Cheshire, Danish blue, or Cheddar with French bread and butter.

And every few months, her chest filled with phlegm. Bouts of coughing degenerated into feeling unable to breathe, and eventually she became bedridden, until antibiotics helped her fight her way back to health. Her mother suffered from the same debilitating bouts of bronchitis and pneumonia, but neither of them linked the problem to anything in the kitchen.

In her twenties, she stopped eating meat for ethical reasons. But her taste for cheese continued. She patronized specialty shops for hard English cheeses and blues and loved their salty scent, carved from a block or sliced for a sandwich. Her respiratory problems continued, too. Every few months, she found herself in bed, unable to work.

One day a friend told her about the source of veal. She already knew that veal calves were raised in tiny boxes and were sometimes rendered anemic so their flesh would remain pale and rubbery. The industry was so cruel that her mother refused to prepare it, even though veal *cordon bleu* was her father's favorite dish. But her friend explained that veal calves come from dairy farms. Cows impregnated to produce milk soon have calves, and male calves become veal. In effect, the friend said, there is a little bit of a veal calf in every glass of milk and every chunk of cheese.

So, that was it. Dairy products had to go, too, she decided. Out with the cheese, out with the condensed milk, out with the lot of it. She stopped buying them and, before long, she didn't miss them anymore.

About a year later, it hit her: Her respiratory problems had gone away. Ever since she had dropped dairy products from her diet, she had not had even one bout of bronchitis. And she learned that many other people had found the same thing.

Respiratory problems can hit anywhere between the lungs and the sinuses, and even the ears. Many young children suffer with otitis media—a painful inflammation of the middle ear that often starts as an upper respiratory infection and congestion in the Eustachian tubes. As middle-ear secretions accumulate, they provide a breeding ground for infections.

Why do dairy proteins trigger these problems? Is it that the human immune system recognizes dairy proteins as foreign and launches an inflammatory assault to try to eliminate them? Inflammation would explain the runny nose and congestion.

In my view, it is still not entirely clear why avoiding dairy products is often so helpful for otitis media or other inflammatory conditions.[8] But the good news is that you do not need to wait for researchers to connect the physiological dots. There is no risk in getting away from dairy products. If you have respiratory problems, going dairy-free is a really good idea. You will soon see what it will do for you.

Tackling Migraines

Lauren was twenty-three when she had her first migraine. It began with just an odd visual phenomenon—her field of vision suddenly narrowed. Then the pain hit. This was not some run-of-the-mill stress headache. This was a sledgehammer. Along with the pain in her head, she was sick—nauseated and vomiting. She could not tolerate light and had to retire to a dark room and wait for the punishment to end.

Terrible as it was, that first migraine was not entirely a surprise; her cousin had them, too. And over the next few months, they happened again and again. Although many people find that their migraines go away with sleep, Lauren's were more persistent. A headache coming on Monday would not go away until after her *second* night's sleep—that is, Wednesday morning. She was a hardworking law student, but when a headache struck, she was unable to study or to do much of anything other than wait for it to go away.

One day, while interviewing for a summer job—one of those all-important placements that law students hope will lead to a career—Lauren was doing her best to impress her future employer with her insightfulness, skill, and resilience when a migraine forced her to excuse herself from the interview to throw up in the bathroom (she did not get the job).

A neurologist prescribed a medication that did seem to knock out her headaches, but she soon found that it really just deferred them—her headaches soon came roaring back. And the medication made her feel physically very odd, as if she were floating. This was not the answer.

What Is a Migraine?

A migraine is not just a bad headache. It is pounding pain, and it lasts for hours. Curiously, it often occurs on just one side of your head, which is where its name comes from (Greek *hemikrania* means "one side of the head.")

The pain is sometimes preceded by an aura of flashing lights, blind spots, or other sensory phenomena—like Lauren's narrowed vision. Along with it, you feel sick. Lights and sounds are hard to take, forcing many migraine sufferers to lie down in a dark room to wait it out.

The diagnosis is usually straightforward. Your doctor will look for the following criteria, which were set by the International Headache Society:

1. Five or more attacks (or just two attacks if accompanied by an aura)
2. A duration of four hours to three days
3. At least two of the following:
   a. One-sided
   b. Pulsating
   c. Moderate to severe intensity

    d. Aggravation by or causing avoidance of routine physical activity
4. One or both of the following:
    a. Nausea and/or vomiting
    b. Sensitivity to both light and sound

Medications can reduce migraine frequency and treat them when they strike, and sometimes they can be lifesavers. As Lauren found, however, their benefit is limited and they have side effects. Also, paradoxically, frequent painkiller use can lead to chronic headaches.

So what causes these horrible headaches? The answer is really not known. Despite the fact that migraines are very common, the mechanism is only vaguely understood as some combination of changes in the blood vessels, brain tissues, and neurotransmitters.

Migraines tend to hit when you are stressed or sleep-deprived, if you have missed a meal, or if you are near your menstrual period. Weather changes and unusual odors can bring them on, too. And food plays a big role.

Cheese is a trigger for many people—especially aged cheese—and it was for Lauren, too. And this was not good. Coming from an Italian family, she loved cannoli (ricotta-stuffed pastry desserts), and ricotta straight out of the package, as well as pizza drowning in mozzarella, mascarpone, plus Brie, Camembert, blue cheese—she loved them all.

Lauren found that a little cottage cheese might be safe, but an expensive aged artisanal cheese that was a cheese maker's pride and joy was certain to incapacitate her. Even a little Parmesan would set off a headache. When she avoided aged cheeses and coffee, her headaches became less frequent. But they were not gone. They continued to arrive every two weeks or so.

Foods and Migraine

What is it about cheese? Why would it trigger migraines? The usual explanation is *tyramine*, a compound found in aged cheeses, as well as in some meats, chocolate, soy sauce, sauerkraut, and other foods. Tyramine is produced from the amino acid *tyrosine*, which is found in each of these foods. During fermentation, the tyrosine turns to tyramine, the presumed migraine culprit.

But tyramine might not be the whole story. Many migraine sufferers find that dairy products in general—including unfermented ones—can tighten the headaches' grip, and many other foods can, too, with considerable variation from one person to another.

In 1983, researchers at London's Hospital for Sick Children tested a special diet for children with migraines. The idea was to eliminate a broad range of common triggers. Amazingly, out of eighty-eight children, seventy-eight recovered completely, and four more were greatly improved.[9] In adults, elimination diets have had somewhat less consistent results, but even so, trigger-free diets help many people—up to about half of the participants in research studies.[10] Avoiding fatty foods helps, too, reducing headache frequency and intensity.[11]

Foods can also help indirectly. Our research team found that a low-fat plant-based diet can have a powerful effect on hormones, reducing menstrual cramps and premenstrual symptoms, as we saw in Chapter 4.[12] And that means that the same diet change should help prevent premenstrual migraines.

Getting Headache-Free

The turning point in Lauren's life came when she heard a radio advertisement for a research study our team was conducting.[13] She came into our center to see what the study was about.

Our goal was to help migraine sufferers identify their dietary triggers and eliminate them. Most had already heard that aged cheese, chocolate, red wine, and processed meats could spark headaches, but there seemed to be other common triggers, too. So we asked the participants to eliminate all the potential trigger foods, using a list we provided. Then, once their headaches were gone or as close to gone as possible, we asked them to return the trigger foods to their diets, one at a time, to see which ones caused headaches and which ones did not.

Lauren jumped in. Over the next two months, her headaches became less and less frequent. And finally they just stopped. The key, she found, was not just avoiding aged cheeses, but all cheeses and other dairy products. It was a little tough at first, but eventually she lost her taste for them. After all, it's hard to love a sledgehammer. Instead of cheese, she found she could add avocado to salads and could bring a savory flavor to pasta with a good olive oil and salt.

Chocolate turned out to be a trigger, too, but not such a harsh one. Lauren found that chocolate could provoke a minor headache, but not a crashing migraine.

Lauren is now migraine-free and feels great. She is married and has a busy job handling complex financial issues on Capitol Hill. Although it is challenging work that could give anyone a headache, Lauren says, "I don't even think about migraines anymore. It's amazing. I feel cured. Now I just don't get headaches."

If you would like to try the same track-down-your-triggers diet that Lauren used, you'll see the details in the Appendix.

Conquering Joint Pain

Could a cheese sandwich make your joints hurt? Arthritis is something we attribute to older age or maybe to genetic traits passed along from our parents. But rheumatoid arthritis is an inflammatory condition—your joints do not just ache; they are also swollen and tender, and that means that something is triggering the attack. And if that is true, it means we should be able to track down the culprit and eliminate it.

Let me share Irene's experience. Irene was a nurse, living in Richmond. She was young and had always been active, but she began to notice pains in her joints. Over time, the pain gradually got worse, and was accompanied by stiffness, especially in the morning. It took her longer and longer to loosen up enough to get around. As time went on, it took a bigger and bigger toll on her life.

"Walking was very difficult. My hips and elbows were killing me. I couldn't pick up my daughter. I just couldn't do the things I wanted to do, and my life was just falling away from me."

Her rheumatologist started her on prednisone, a steroid that alleviates symptoms but has so many side effects—insomnia, digestive problems, and weight gain, among others—that no one would want to remain on it longer than necessary. The doctor then wrote her a prescription for methotrexate, a drug typically used for cancer chemotherapy that is now commonly used for arthritis. It has side effects, too. This is not to say that these drugs should never be used. They have actually helped many people. But even with drug treatments, Irene was still hurting. And she wanted to get at the *cause* of her problem.

Searching on the Internet, she found information about foods and joint pain. Specifically, she learned that a plant-based diet could help. She presented the idea to her rheumatologist, who turned out to be less than enthusiastic about it. "He said, basically, 'you're insane,'" she remembers. But even without his support, she decided to change her diet. What did she have to lose?

Quickly, she began to feel better. Bit by bit, her pain started to disappear. Before long, she was able to walk without pain or stiffness. And she was able to ride a bike, and eventually able to jump on her backyard trampoline. This was not the picture of a pain-ridden arthritis patient. Irene was feeling better than she had in years.

"The minute you can be pain free, it just gives you a whole other outlook on life. You wouldn't believe that food can make that type of a difference in your life. And it does. I have my life back. I have a good life. I'm so thankful for what I have."

Let's also meet Karen. She was forty-seven, living in Ohio, when she started to experience pain and stiffness in her neck. We all have a little stiffness from time to time—from over-exercising or sleeping in a wrong position—but this was different.

Although aches and pains come and go, her neck pain was gradually worsening. When she tried to drive, she was unable to look around to change lanes and had to have someone with her to check for traffic. As time went on, the pain radiated down her arms all the way to her fingertips.

She saw her doctor, who ordered an MRI and took a good hard look at her bones and joints. She had seriously inflamed vertebrae that would drastically reduce her ability to move. Luckily, there was a treatment that might work. The operation would cost $50,000, but her doctor was ready to schedule it, and her insurance company was ready to write the check. And maybe that would be best, it seemed, because life was becoming unlivable.

But Karen then saw a new doctor who encouraged her to first try a diet change. Aiming to reduce her inflammation and allow her body to heal, he advised getting away from dairy products.

And while she was at it, why not get all animal products out of her diet? She did, and within a week, she began to feel better. The pain started to subside. Within two months, it was gone. Since then she has not needed anything for pain—not an aspirin or ibuprofen or anything else. The stiffness and immobility are gone, and she never needed the surgery that had been recommended. And oddly enough, her insurance company, which had been ready to spend $50,000 on surgery, refused to cover the cost of her nutrition consultation.

Fighting Arthritis with Food

Arthritis comes in many forms. *Osteoarthritis* is a common condition usually attributed to wear and tear on joint cartilage and bone. *Rheumatoid arthritis* is an autoimmune disorder, meaning that the body is making antibodies that are attacking the body's own tissues. It causes inflammation in the joints of the hands and feet, eventually working its way to the wrists, elbows, shoulders, ankles, knees, and hips. The joints are tender and swollen, and often stiff in the morning. Psoriatic (pronounced sore-*EE-attic*) arthritis is a condition of painful joints that sometimes comes along with scaly, itchy skin, a condition called *psoriasis.*

If you have rheumatoid arthritis, psoriasis, psoriatic arthritis, or any kind of inflammatory condition, run—don't walk—to a dairy-free, plant-based diet. Researchers have long known that these conditions follow a geographic pattern—they were historically rare in Japan and China, and common in Europe and North America.[14] Geographic differences often reflect diet differences. You would not find much cheesecake in Japan and China, at least not traditionally. That goes for dairy products in general. They were not part of the culture until Westernization introduced them in the past few decades. And in Asia, just as in Western countries, psoriasis is becoming more common as our collective diet worsens over time.[15]

Researchers have long noted that foods contribute to rheumatoid arthritis and that diet changes can help. Back in 1991, researchers in Norway tested a dairy-free and meat-free diet in a group of people suffering from rheumatoid arthritis. Within a month, participants found that their joint swelling and tenderness had improved and their morning stiffness was better. Blood tests confirmed that, indeed, their inflammation was subsiding.[16] Other studies have shown similar benefits.[17] Dr. John McDougall found that inflammation can improve within just four weeks on a low-fat, dairy-free, vegan diet. Pain, stiffness, joint swelling, and tenderness all improved.[18]

Psoriatic Arthritis

"Psoriatic arthritis" became a household word when star golfer Phil Mickelson came down with it just before the 2010 U.S. Open. It started as pain near his ankle, making it hard to walk. And then his left index finger and right wrist felt like they had been sprained. At first, he attributed the pain to years of practice, and he hoped it would soon pass. But one day, his joint pain was so intense he could barely get out of bed.

With the help of a rheumatologist, he was able to get back on his feet. He then decided to see if a diet change would help him fend off future attacks. He announced to his golf buddies and the press that he was going vegetarian.

"What!?" In the conservative world of golf, where clothing styles and club membership rules are updated begrudgingly, steak, beer, diabetes, and heart disease are all normal fare on a golf course. A vegetarian diet—that's something new. It did not help that Phil Mickelson is part-owner of the Five Guys burger chain.

His not-so-healthful food tastes, aided and abetted by less-than-supportive comments from sports reporters, meant that his dietary resolve was not what it might have been. He ended up signing on as a spokesperson for *Enbrel*, the $30,000-a-year injectable that works by partially disabling the immune system. It does indeed mute the autoimmune attack on the joints, but also leaves you susceptible to dangerous infections, including tuberculosis, as you'll hear in the manufacturer's television advertisements.

Tackling Tendonitis

While we're looking at orthopedic problems, foods may also affect your tendons—those fibrous bands that connect your muscles to your bones—like the Achilles tendon that attaches your calf muscle to your heel. When they become inflamed, the condition is called *tendonitis.*

The problem is usually chalked up to overuse. But something else is clearly afoot. First of all, people with diabetes are prone to tendonitis, which suggests that something about body chemistry is contributing to the problem. Second, researchers from Australia's Monash University found a link with cholesterol, finding that people with tendon problems generally have more "bad cholesterol" (that is, low-density lipoprotein, or LDL, cholesterol) in their bloodstreams.[19] They also have less "good cholesterol" (high-density lipoprotein, or HDL, cholesterol).

You already know that cheese is the mother lode of the fat and cholesterol that can increase "bad cholesterol" levels in the blood, and it appears that, just as unhealthful cholesterol levels can contribute to heart disease, they are also associated with tendon problems.

No one knows more about tendonitis than David Carter. In

2014, he was a 285-pound pro football player, and he was hurting. His tendonitis was so bad that he could barely lift himself out of the bathtub. One day, watching a documentary about nutrition and health, he learned that dairy products might be part of the problem. In other words, some of the very foods he had been eating to bulk up might have contributed to inflammation. So he scrapped them. He adopted an entirely vegan diet, and his life transformed. Within two months, his pain was gone. His speed and strength improved. And then, his only problem was maintaining a linebacker's weight on the world's most effective slimming diet!

In 2016, the Green Bay Packers quarterback Aaron Rodgers announced that he was eliminating cheese from his diet. What would make the Cheeseheads' favorite athlete dump dairy? "I just wanted to get healthier," he said. At age thirty-two, Rodgers was eager to extend his career, and cutting out dairy products was part of his healthy eating plan.

"Through your eating, you can reduce inflammation," he said. "And with a knee condition I've had a long time, it really started after the surgery, thinking about exactly what I'm going to eat the first couple of weeks after surgery to kind of limit the amount of inflammation in my knee and carried that around the rest of the offseason."[20]

Healthy Skin

What about your skin? If cheese and other dairy products can affect your lungs, brain, and joints, could they also inflame your skin? Could they contribute to acne? Let me share Amy's story with you.

When Amy was five years old, she thought she was dying,

and so did her doctors. Three days earlier, her family had bought her a Happy Meal at a McDonald's in Pittsburgh. The symptoms started within hours—dizziness, nausea, and diarrhea—and they worsened quickly. Her parents rushed her to the emergency room, and she was admitted to the hospital. But, despite good care, she went downhill fast.

The disease was hemolytic-uremic syndrome, caused by a cattle-born bacterial infection that, years later, became famous when children eating at a Seattle-area Jack in the Box became ill. In the massive outbreak, more than a hundred people were hospitalized and four children died.

The disease was all but unknown when Amy was hospitalized in Pittsburgh. As her kidneys failed, she needed dialysis, and was put on the list for a transplant. One day, she overheard her doctors saying she was not likely to survive.

But she did survive. It took three months, but she eventually improved enough to leave the hospital.

Not long afterward, her father took the family on a drive through the Pennsylvania countryside. It was good to be outside, to smell the fresh air, and to cruise through the fields and forests.

Rounding a corner, her father suddenly slammed on his brakes. A cow was crossing the road, and they were inches from an accident. They slowly crept around the cow and safely continued their journey. But in the ensuing discussion, five-year-old Amy thought about how a cow had almost died, just as she herself had almost died. And she thought about how that cow was destined to turn into hamburger, and that wasn't good for anybody. And that day, she made a very grown-up decision to stop eating meat.

That was a good move, except that removing meat meant

replacing it with a lot of equally unhealthful things. "I was eating pizza all the time, with extra cheese," she said. "And lots of Doritos and junk food."

And she did not feel well. When her periods started at age twelve, her flow was unusually heavy and lasted two to three weeks at a time. She developed menstrual migraines. And she had problems with her complexion. Acne is common in adolescence, of course. But for Amy, it was worse. "I had terrible acne all over my face, and it went down my shoulders and back."

At age fourteen, she made another decision. Out with the cheese, milk, and all other dairy products, and in with soy milk and rice milk. She topped her pizza with veggies and tomato sauce, instead of cheese. Although cheese cravings called out to her for a week or two, she ignored them. "Within a few weeks, everything started to change," she said. Her skin cleared up. Her bloating and other symptoms were gone. "It was astounding."

Today, she still likes cheese, but that means cashew cheese or vegan mac and cheese, instead of the animal-derived varieties. Her four-year-old daughter has never tasted meat, cheese, or any other animal product, and has been in perfect health. "The change was a little tough at first, but worth it," Amy said.

Dairy Products and Acne

Until fairly recently, most experts discounted the role of foods in acne. It's not cheese, chocolate, or grease that causes pimples, they said. The problem is hormones. And true enough, hormone shifts contribute to breakouts.

But a new view came from studies of traditional cultures. The islanders of Papua New Guinea, the Aché of Paraguay, the Inuits of northern Canada, and Okinawans prior to World War

II—all were more or less free of acne as long as their traditional diets held. And when diets were Westernized—or "modernized"—to include cheeseburgers and pizza, acne became a common problem.[21]

In 2005, Harvard researchers asked more than 47,000 nurses about what they had eaten as adolescents and whether they had experienced acne as teenagers.[22] Crunching the numbers, it turned out that chocolate got a not-guilty verdict. Ditto for soda, French fries, and pizza. The food that lit up in the statistics was milk. The milk drinkers had more acne, and how much of a problem it was depended on the fat content. Those who drank the most whole milk were about 12 percent more likely to have had severe acne. But those who drank the most *skim* milk were *44 percent* more likely to have had severe acne. In other words, fatty milk was a problem, but low-fat milk seemed to be a much worse problem.

The researchers realized that some people's memories might have been a bit faulty when it came to the details of their diets as adolescents. So they did a new study that addressed the issues more directly. They followed 4,273 boys and 6,094 girls, aged nine to fifteen, over a three-year period, watching their food intake and whether they developed acne or not. The results mirrored those of the earlier study. The more milk the children drank, the more likely they were to have acne. And skim milk was implicated at least as much as whole milk.[23] Skim is much lower in fat, obviously. But it is higher in both protein and sugar (lactose).

So, yes, although the fat in milk might lead to weight gain and all manner of other problems, for acne, the main suspect was milk protein.

The science of food and acne is still in its infancy. But the common experience of people who have dumped dairy and found that their skin improved suggests that going dairy-free is well worth a try.

Better Digestion

So far, we have looked at asthma and other respiratory problems, allergies, headaches, joint pains, and skin problems and how they can improve dramatically when people ditch the cheese and other dairy products. And there is another part of the body that merits attention in this chapter: our oft-tortured digestive tracts.

Ann Wheat grew up in a dairying family. Her father was a milk processor. As cans of milk arrived, he turned it into whipping cream, strawberry and chocolate milk, and ice cream sundaes. Ann was the "soda jerk," making milkshakes and ice cream cones in the summertime.

But Ann was not healthy. As a child, she had respiratory problems, including a serious bout of pneumonia. She had earaches and sore throats and needed a tonsillectomy at age five. It never occurred to anyone that dairy proteins might be contributing to the inflammation in her ears, throat, and lungs. When doctors diagnosed anemia, none suggested that perhaps dairy products might be reducing this little girl's ability to absorb iron.

Worst of all, she had chronic digestive problems. During her toddler years, her mother and grandmother—both nurses—worried about her severe constipation. When she was eight, continuing digestive disorders led her grandmother to take her to the Mayo Clinic. But X-rays and blood samples turned up nothing. Try a psychiatrist, the doctors suggested.

Although researchers have long known that dairy products can contribute to constipation in young children, many pediatricians have somehow missed this message.[24] Not until Ann was forty-two did a doctor suggest eliminating dairy products. And as soon as she did, her digestive problems became a thing of the past.

"Why hadn't someone come to this conclusion before?" she asked. "It would have saved me years of pain and suffering, and I would not have had to watch in frustrated agony as my own child suffered with the same problems."

Like so many others who have discovered the answer to health problems, she felt strongly motivated to share what she had found. Along with her husband Larry, Ann helped launch a restaurant called Millennium that served dairy-free vegan dinners and quickly became a San Francisco legend.

"I wish this message could be shared with everyone. I hate to see others suffer, especially children. Dairy products should come with warning labels."

Preventing Type 1 Diabetes

Type 1 diabetes is a condition in which the pancreas no longer makes insulin, the hormone that moves glucose (sugar) from the bloodstream into the cells of the body. Without insulin, glucose builds up in the blood. Usually diagnosed in childhood or early adulthood, the disease increases the risk of heart disease, visual impairment, loss of kidney function, amputations, and other serious problems. Insulin injections are essential for bringing it under control.

For many years, researchers have known that infants consuming cow's milk formula have a higher risk of developing diabetes, compared with breast-fed babies. Presumably, the baby's immune system recognizes cow's milk proteins as foreign and reacts by producing antibodies against them. These antibodies, in turn, inadvertently attack the baby's own pancreas, killing off the insulin-producing cells.

In 1992, the *New England Journal of Medicine* reported the results of tests on 142 children newly diagnosed with type 1 diabetes.[25] Every single child had antibodies against cow's milk proteins. In further tests, a portion of the cow's milk protein turned out to be a biochemical match for a protein in the insulin-producing pancreas cells. So antibodies against milk would, in theory at least, be primed to attack and destroy these cells—a disastrous case of "friendly fire."

A pilot study looked to see if avoiding cow's milk formula might prevent type 1 diabetes. It included 242 newborns who were deemed to be at risk for diabetes (each had a first-degree relative with the condition). Researchers encouraged their mothers to breast-feed and then, when the mothers were ready to transition their infants to the bottle, the researchers asked half to use a special formula in which dairy proteins were broken up into individual amino acids. The other half were to use a regular cow's milk formula.[26] Following the children through their first six to eight years of life, the modified formula did indeed appear to have some benefit in reducing diabetes risk. As of this writing, however, the full test results are not yet in.

That said, my impression is that we need to go much further. This pilot study restricted dairy consumption only during the first several months of life, and it did not ask breast-feeding mothers to avoid cow's milk in their own diets. So the mothers were still delivering traces of cow's milk proteins to their infants every time they breast-fed and giving their children dairy products later on.

If dairy proteins are a culprit in type 1 diabetes, the way to avoid them is to (1) steer clear of dairy products throughout childhood, and (2) ask mothers to avoid dairy products while they are breast-feeding so as to avoid passing dairy proteins to their children through breast milk. And cheese is at the top of the list of products to avoid, because it has particularly concentrated milk proteins. There is no risk to avoiding it and, potentially, great benefit.

Unmasking the Culprits

As we have seen, cheese contributes to a striking range of health problems. Although this chapter has covered many serious health issues, among the most important are those we will tackle in the next chapter, when we look at the surprising and confusing issues caused by the fat and cholesterol found in every slice of cheese.

CHAPTER 6

Heart Disease, Diabetes, and the French Paradox

At the time, weighing 285 pounds wasn't entirely a bad thing.

Marc Ramirez was born in McAllen, Texas, near the Mexican border. When he was seven, his mother divorced her drug-dealing husband, then eventually moved the family to a new home north of Chicago.

Money was tight, and their diet was not as healthful as it might have been. "My mother got government aid. And I remember those five-pound blocks of cheese," he said. "We drenched food in it. We put it all over tortillas, enchiladas, and tacos. We put it in quesadillas. We didn't know better." That, along with other dietary issues, meant that Marc gained quite a lot of weight.

By the time he finished high school, Marc weighed 285 pounds. On his six-foot, two-inch frame, that meant he was well into the obese range. That would be of concern in just about any other circumstance. But Marc was tough and had learned how to play serious football. So the University of Michigan—one of the top college football teams in the nation—recruited him with an all-expenses-paid scholarship. Marc played right guard, meaning his job was to tear holes in the opponents' defenses and get his runners through.

He kept up his weight with pizza, burgers, steak, and fried chicken. Vegetables were afterthoughts. "If I ever had a salad, I drowned it in ranch dressing."

After college, the inevitable happened. He developed type 2 diabetes. He also had high cholesterol, high blood pressure, heartburn, psoriasis, and erectile dysfunction. The weight that had helped him smash a defensive line had turned against him. His health, his energy, and even his sexual function had all gone to pot.

He knew all about diabetes. His mother suffered with it; by the time she died at age sixty-one, she had endured heart surgery and had severe visual problems and failing kidneys. His youngest brother had lost his vision, his kidney function, and his right leg to the disease. His twin brother had diabetes, too, as did two sisters.

"When I was diagnosed, I was thinking about what had happened to my mother and my little brother," he said. "I saw myself going down the same path. And I remembered how each of us was called into the doctor's office to see if we could donate a kidney to my mother. I decided I did not want to put my family in that predicament. And years from now, I don't want to have family visiting me in a nursing home; I want to be with them on the soccer field."

But on his cheese- and meat-heavy diet, things were not going well. He took oral diabetes medications, plus twice-daily insulin injections, along with pills to control his cholesterol and blood pressure. "I asked my doctor if I could ever get off the shots. But he explained that I needed insulin to protect my organs, and that I would be on it for the rest of my life."

Understanding Diabetes

Diabetes means there is too much sugar—glucose—in the bloodstream. In the last chapter, we looked at type 1 diabetes and how dairy proteins might play a role in destroying the insulin-producing cells of the pancreas. In the much more common form—type 2—the pancreas still makes insulin, but the cells of the body do not respond to it normally. And when insulin cannot get glucose into the cells, it builds up in the bloodstream.

Abundant scientific evidence shows that a key contributor to this breakdown of insulin function is fat. Microscopic particles of fat building up *inside muscle and liver cells* stop insulin from working properly. This process occurs amazingly quickly. In controlled tests, researchers have infused fat mixtures into the bloodstreams of volunteers, causing insulin to sputter and fail within just a few hours.[1] Luckily, that process is reversible, but we are getting ahead of ourselves. *Saturated fat* (the kind that is prevalent in cheese and meat) appears to be more disruptive of insulin function than unsaturated fats (the kind in vegetable oils).[2]

You don't have to have an intravenous fat infusion to get diabetes. You can do the same thing with fatty foods. Cheese has plenty of fat, as you know only too well, and people who eat cheese and other fatty foods are at much higher risk of developing diabetes, compared with people who avoid them.

Reversing Diabetes

Marc took his problems seriously. He dieted. He counted calories and ramped up his exercise. But the results were meager. After lots of attempts, he realized that losing weight was not so easy.

Then, in 2011, he learned about a completely different approach. Instead of calorie-counting, the idea was to avoid animal products.

By knocking out the animal fat and cholesterol, he had a chance at good health.

Our research team had pioneered this method, finding that diabetes often improves dramatically and sometimes even goes away. It makes sense: If fat particles inside the cells gum up insulin's ability to function, what could be better than skipping animal fats altogether and giving the cells a chance to clean themselves up? It also proved powerful for improving body weight, cholesterol, and blood pressure.

Marc and his wife, Kim, decided to give it a try. Out with the cheese, out with the meat. They resolved to eat healthful foods from now on. Although it took a while for it to become second nature, it wasn't difficult, and they found plenty of healthful, appealing foods.

"Our breakfast would be oatmeal topped with cinnamon, bananas, and sliced pecans or walnuts," he said. "For lunch, we'd have bean burritos and burrito bowls, black bean tacos, stir-fries, or veggie fajitas. Dessert could be a fruit medley with bananas, strawberries, and blueberries, or maybe a chocolate nirvana shake as a treat." They found many books, websites, and other resources, and as time went on, they found it easier and easier to find the healthful foods they were looking for. "It's simple," he said. "We can eat anywhere."

The results came fast. "In three months, I lost 50 pounds, and my blood sugars plummeted." Cholesterol-lowering medication had already reduced his cholesterol to 164. But twenty-six days of a plant-based diet dropped it all the way to 104. His LDL ("bad") cholesterol fell from 87 to 44. His triglycerides went from 191 to 111. "In less than two months, I was off my insulin and all four diabetes medications. I had been taking lisinopril for my blood pressure and a simvastatin for my cholesterol, and my doctor stopped everything. He said, 'You are my star patient!'"

The heartburn, psoriasis, and erectile dysfunction all disappeared. "I was a new man," he said. And he has inspired his family. His daughter graduated from the University of Michigan and is now a third-grade teacher. His son is at the university now. And slowly but surely, they saw the value of the diet changes their parents made, and have changed their own diets.

And all that cheese and steak—does Marc miss them? "This will sound surprising," he said. "But now those foods gross me out. They remind me of being overweight and sick. I don't miss them at all."

Cheese and Heart Disease

Throwing out the cheese and other animal products does more than tackle diabetes. It also has a powerful effect on heart disease. In 1990, Dr. Dean Ornish published the results of a landmark study.[3] He had asked a group of heart patients to begin a low-fat vegetarian diet, along with other healthy lifestyle changes—modest exercise, stress reduction, and avoiding smoking. A year later, he measured the plaques in their coronary arteries with an *angiogram*—a special X-ray of the heart—and compared the findings to the same test done at the beginning of the study.

The results made medical history. The patients' narrowed arteries had begun to reopen—so much so that there was a measurable difference in 82 percent of the participants in the first year. Until then, most doctors had assumed that heart disease was irreversible. But with the right kind of diet and lifestyle, patients have power they never had before. They can cut their cholesterol, blood pressure, and body weight, reopen their arteries, and dramatically reduce the chances they will ever have a heart attack.[4]

Let me share a few essentials on heart disease:

Common heart disease occurs when cholesterol particles in the bloodstream work their way into the artery wall and form *plaques*—bumps made of fat, cholesterol, and overgrowing muscle cells that narrow the passageway for blood. A plaque can break open like a blister. When it does, it can trigger the formation of a blood clot like a cork in the artery. Blood flow stops. And without a blood supply, a portion of the heart muscle dies, in what is called a *myocardial infarction*, or a heart attack.

Where are all these cholesterol particles coming from? A fair number come from your plate. Dairy products, meat, and eggs contain cholesterol, and much of it passes into your bloodstream, adding to the cholesterol that is already there. More importantly, the *saturated* ("bad") fat in dairy products and meats increases the amount of cholesterol in your blood.

If you were to set aside animal products—cheese, meat, and all the rest—you would have very little saturated fat and effectively no cholesterol on your plate, and your cholesterol level would likely plummet.

Your Body Makes All the Cholesterol You Need

Your body normally makes tiny amounts of cholesterol, which serves several functions. First, cholesterol particles maintain your cells' flexibility. Think of them like little hinges in your cell membranes. Your body also uses cholesterol as a raw material for building hormones—testosterone, estrogens, and others—and the bile acids that help you digest food. So your body is always making a little bit of cholesterol for these needs.

But here's the key: Your body makes all the cholesterol you need. If you eat foods that contain cholesterol or that harbor the fats that increase the amount of cholesterol in your bloodstream, you end up with more cholesterol in your blood than you need and you are at higher risk of health problems.

So, getting rid of meats, dairy products, and fatty foods in general is a good idea. But how bad is cheese, really? Is it really going to put my ticker at risk?

Well, have a look at what is in a typical 2-ounce serving of cheese—the amount a person might put on a sandwich:

First, fat: Saturated fat raises blood cholesterol levels, and cheese and other dairy products are the biggest source of saturated fat in the American diet, as you'll see in the figure below. A 2-ounce sandwich-sized serving of Cheddar has as much saturated ("bad") fat as *eight* slices of bacon (11 grams).[5]

In case you were wondering, goat cheese is no better. In fact, part of the reason some people choose it is that it has a mouthfeel that is a bit fattier than cow's milk varieties. Look up semi-soft goat cheese on the USDA's website, and you'll find that 2 ounces have 12 grams of saturated fat. If it's hard goat cheese, that number is close to 14 grams. That's like eating eight sausage links.

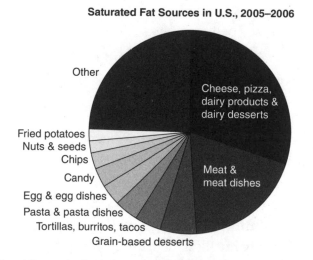

Saturated Fat Sources in U.S., 2005–2006

Source: National Cancer Institute. Sources of saturated fat in the diets of the U.S. population ages 2 years and older, NHANES 2005–2006. Risk Factor Monitoring and Methods. Cancer Control and Population Sciences. http://riskfactor.cancer.gov/diet /food sources/sat_fat/sf.html. Accessed November 14, 2015.

Second, cholesterol: That 2-ounce Cheddar serving also packs 56 milligrams of cholesterol.[6] That is as much or more than you'll find in typical meats.

Third, sodium: Sodium raises blood pressure, which, in turn, increases your risk of heart disease. You'll remember from Chapter 1 that salt is essential to the cheese-making process. Cheese makers use lots and lots of it. Here are the numbers:

For comparison, a medium-sized apple has 1 milligram of sodium. An orange has 2. A potato has 13, until it is turned into salted potato chips, in which case a 2-ounce serving has 330 milligrams. And, as we saw in Chapter 2, 2 ounces of Cheddar or Muenster pack more than 350 milligrams, and Velveeta has a whopping *800 milligrams of sodium*—ready to raise your blood pressure, overwork your heart, and contribute to heart failure.

Fatty foods like cheese also make the blood "thicker"—that is, more viscous—and it requires more effort for the heart and blood vessels to move that thicker blood along. As a result, your blood pressure rises.

So, yes, cheese spells trouble.

Bad for the Heart, Bad for the Brain

So fatty, high-cholesterol foods are bad for your heart and increase your diabetes risk. But they may do something even worse. As we get older, many people succumb to Alzheimer's disease, losing their ability to reason, remember, and function from day to day. In 1993, the Chicago Health and Aging Project set out to see if this devastating problem might have any links to foods. Carefully tracking the eating habits of a large group of volunteers, the researchers then waited to see who developed Alzheimer's disease and who remained clear.

Ten years later, they reported a striking finding. The same

"bad fat" (saturated fat) that is implicated in heart disease was also linked to Alzheimer's disease. Specifically, those who ate the most saturated fat (think cheese, meat, etc., on a daily basis) had two to three times the risk, compared with those who indulged less often in these products.[7]

Researchers in Finland looked at milder memory problems and found a similar connection with "bad fat." In a group of 1,341 adults, those who had the most saturated fat in their diets were more than twice as likely to develop memory problems in old age, compared with those consuming less.[8]

Why would cheese and similar foods be linked to Alzheimer's disease? The reason might be cholesterol. Researchers at Kaiser Permanente tracked cholesterol levels in 9,844 Kaiser members, finding that the higher a person's cholesterol, the more likely he or she was to develop Alzheimer's disease.[9] Cholesterol seems to play a role in brain changes, just as it does in heart disease.

Other factors play important roles in brain problems, too. Trans fats—the kind found in doughnuts and other snack foods—are linked to Alzheimer's disease, just as saturated fat is. And certain things are protective: vitamin E–rich foods and exercise, in particular. If you are interested in more details, let me invite you to look at my previous book, *Power Foods for the Brain*.

Industry Fights Back Again...

The food industry has not sat still for criticism. It has found elaborate ways to do damage control for the reputations of cheese and other unhealthful foods. Because industry myths have pervaded the media and popular understanding, I would like to take a bit of time to help you sort things out, starting with one of the nutrition world's favorite myths...

The French Paradox

Oh, la la! People in France eat a lot of cheese, butter, and cream, but they have an enviably low risk of heart disease. Let's dig in!

The term "French Paradox" was coined in 1986 by the Organisation Internationale de la Vigne et du Vin—the French winegrowers—and the statistics were impressive: In France, heart disease deaths occurred at one-quarter the rate in Britain.[10] The take-home message was as clear as a price tag in a gourmet food shop: Whatever dangers cheese or cream might throw at you, a bottle of French wine will protect you. The French Paradox was the darling of the producers of wine, cheese, and every other product in need of redemption.

The French were indeed drinking a lot of wine. Or rather, French wine drinkers tended to put away a lot more of it, compared with wine drinkers in Britain—the 1988 figures were 13.1 liters per person per year in France, compared with 8.5 liters in Britain.[11] And the French love cheese—Emmental, Camembert, Brie, Roquefort, and many, many more.

But cheese and statistics have holes, and we are about to find them. Almost immediately after the idea was floated it started to run aground. The first problem was that French medical authorities handled their statistics differently. A death from *ischemic heart disease*—the common form of heart disease that leads to heart attacks—is called just that in Britain. But in France, it would have been classified as a death from unknown or unspecified causes.[12]

The second issue was smoking. When the "paradox" idea began in the late 1980s, relatively few French women smoked (9 percent), compared with British women (30 percent). That difference gave French women a big advantage in heart health that had nothing to do with wine, cheese, or anything else. For men, smoking rates were similar between the two countries.

But the biggest issue, according to researchers at the Royal London School of Medicine and Dentistry, was the fact that the French diet has changed over time.[13] In 1988, France and Britain looked to have pretty similar diets. Animal fat accounted for 25.7 percent of calories in France, and 27.0 percent in Britain. But a closer look showed that the French had only just gotten to that higher number. In preceding years, animal fat intake was considerably lower, and the lower heart disease rates in France simply reflected the fact that their heart risks had not yet caught up with their worsening diet.

In fact, there really is not a single "French diet." French food habits are heavily influenced by regional traditions. You have no doubt heard of the idea that northern Europe cooks in butter, while southern Europe uses olive oil. But the differences run much deeper and the map is more complicated.

On a French website devoted to women's issues, one woman wrote that, when she was growing up in southern France, vegetables were king. Every meal included three or four different vegetables, and soup was part of every evening meal. Meat was served only in small quantities, except when entertaining guests. When she married a man from Lorraine in northeastern France, she was stunned by how he ate. Dinners focused on *la charcuterie*—that is, pork. "It took me years to convince him to limit it," she wrote.[14]

Another woman responded with exactly the same experience. "What you wrote amused me very much," she said. "Growing up in the country, we had soup every night and meat only once or twice a week." But when she married a man from Lorraine—just like the first woman—"I was shocked to find that his family *ate meat* twice *a day*, with lots of pork dishes." In Britain or America, of course, having meat twice a day has long been the norm.

France has enjoyed Mediterranean traditions in the south, with Italian influences coming from the southeast and Spanish influences from the southwest, along with African foods making the short trip from Algeria and Morocco. Northern and eastern France has been influenced by the traditions of Germany, Switzerland, Holland, and Belgium.

So not only was there not a single "French diet," but in some parts of France, meat was a rarity. So to the extent there was less heart disease in France, it was not likely to be due to cheese being harmless or wine being beneficial. Rather, most French people had not been scarfing down so much animal fat until rather recently, and their heart statistics had not yet caught up to those of their longtime fat-eating counterparts in the U.K.[15]

French Women Actually Do Get Fat

By the way, the changes in eating habits over time have led to obesity in France, just like everywhere else. In a 2009 survey conducted by TNS Sofres Healthcare and the Swiss pharmaceuticals company Roche, 26 percent of women in France were overweight, and another 15 percent were obese. Ditto for men: 39 percent were overweight, and 14 percent were obese.

Although Mireille Guiliano contended in her 2004 book that *French Women Don't Get Fat*, French women have been gradually putting on the kilos. A 2009 study showed that, over the preceding twelve years, the average French person gained more than 3 kilograms—about 7 pounds—and about 5 centimeters (2 inches) around the waist.[16]

It appears that France suffers from heart disease, just like other diseases related to cheese and other dairy products.

Eat Butter?

The French Paradox was an especially memorable bit of nutritional mythology. But it was by no means the last. On June 23, 2014, *Time* magazine's cover proclaimed, in large type, "Eat Butter," and featured a big artistic swirl of the stuff. Several other publications—the *New York Times*, the *Wall Street Journal*, the *New Scientist*, and others—ran similar stories. The experts have been wrong all this time, the articles exclaimed. Fat isn't unhealthy after all. Steak and pork chops won't hurt you. Go ahead, dig in!

Some of the articles were based on a book, *The Big Fat Surprise: Why Butter, Meat and Cheese Belong in a Healthy Diet*. Its author, Nina Teicholz, was on an inexplicably passionate mission to defend butter, meat, and cheese. And she started with Eskimo and Inuit populations of the far north. They have almost no heart disease, she held, despite a diet heavy on fish and blubber. Ergo, fat won't hurt you.

It turns out she was wrong. A study from the University of Ottawa Heart Institute, published in the *Canadian Journal of Cardiology*, showed that cardiovascular disease was at least as frequent among northern native populations as for people in other areas.[17] Strokes have been particularly common, and life expectancy overall was about a decade shorter than for other people. Heart disease had *seemed* rare among northern native populations mainly because reporting of medical problems in general has been spotty.

Teicholz then invoked the Maasai, an African population that is supposedly free of heart disease, despite a diet of meat, milk, and blood.

Again, she was wrong. Researcher George V. Mann wrote in

1978, "We have collected hearts and aortae from 50 authenti-cated Maasai men who died of trauma and we found extensive atherosclerosis."[18] That is, they had serious heart disease.

Okay, so the Maasai's arteries are clogged with atherosclerotic plaques. But they don't have heart attacks, Teicholz maintained; so meat and milk must be safe.

Once again, the argument was DOA. Plaques that form in arteries can rupture, as we saw earlier. When that happens, they spark the formation of clots that block blood flow and cause heart attacks. Teicholz's notion was that the Maasai have plaques, but the plaques somehow never rupture, like time bombs that never explode. This is highly unlikely. A better explanation for the lack of reported heart attacks among the Maasai comes from their tragically short life expectancy. If life is cut short in one's forties by an accident or an infection, plaques have not had enough time to rupture. Moreover, in a rural population with limited medical care and poor medical records, heart attacks may not be recognized or reported. The notion of eating foods that cause atherosclerotic plaques and then hoping they will never explode is simply playing with fire. It is absurdly risky.

Ancel Keys and the Seven Countries Study

Those seeking to make grease look good especially targeted Ancel Keys, the famed University of Minnesota researcher who identified the dangers of fatty foods in the 1950s. Looking at six countries with reliable dietary and medical records, Keys found a clear association between fat intake and heart disease deaths.[19]

University of California at Berkeley statistician Jacob Yerush-almy pointed out that if Keys had zeroed in on more countries than just six, the relationship between saturated fat and heart disease would look weaker.[20] True enough. Including additional countries did muddy the correlation between fat and heart disease deaths, because many of these countries had poor data on diet or medical care at that time. Even so, the correlation between fat and heart deaths remained high, and the correlation between animal protein and heart deaths was even higher.

Playing with Statistics

What really grabbed the headlines, however, was a meta-analysis published in early 2014 by the *Annals of Internal Medicine*.[21] The meta-analysis combined seventy-two smaller studies, finding no overall effect of saturated fat on heart risks. According to the fat lobby, that proved that "bad fat" isn't bad for your heart after all.

A closer look shows something very different. Meta-analyses combine data from many different studies. When these studies use similar methods, combining them makes sense. But when they use very different methods, combining them leads to confusion.

One of the studies in the *Annals* meta-analysis was the Oxford Vegetarian Study,[22] which included 11,000 people whose diets ranged from vegan to ovo-lacto vegetarian to meat-eater, with saturated fat intake ranging from a low of 6 percent of calories to more than 13 percent of calories. The study found that the fattiest diets tripled the risk of dying of heart disease, compared with diets that had very little saturated fat.

But the meta-analysis also included a Swedish study in which *no* groups were on lower-fat diets; all of the study groups averaged more than 13 percent of their calories from saturated fat. Not surprisingly, the study could not identify any effect of avoiding saturated fat, because no groups in the study had a low fat intake.[23]

When the studies were combined, the not-so-well-done studies tended to cancel out the better-quality studies. This certainly does not mean that "bad fat" is suddenly safe.

Cholesterol Confusion

Okay, one last bit of myth-busting, this one related to cholesterol. Specifically, does cholesterol in foods really matter? Yes, there is a lot of it in cheese, but can it actually hurt us?

In 2015, the Dietary Guidelines Advisory Committee, which had the job of revising America's healthy food guidelines, declared that cholesterol in foods poses no risks. Suddenly, newspapers everywhere proclaimed that indulgence was the order of the day. The *Chicago Tribune* wrote:

> The nation's top nutrition advisory panel has dropped charges against dietary cholesterol, recommending that it can no longer be considered a "nutrient of concern." The new thinking: scarfing down cholesterol-chocked delicacies does not appear to significantly affect the level of cholesterol in the blood for many people.[24]

In the *New York Times*, Mark Bittman wrote:

> It finally says that dietary cholesterol isn't much of a problem; you can forget counting milligrams. Think of all those eggs you missed![25]

The public ate up the news. A Gallup poll later that year showed that many apparently agreed that there is no need to try to eat healthfully. Compared with the previous year, the number of Americans avoiding dietary fat had dropped from 56 percent to 47 percent, and the number avoiding excess salt had dropped from 46 percent to 39 percent. What the heck, just eat whatever you want. Food doesn't matter. Cholesterol, fat, and salt can't hurt you.

If you saw these news stories and bought the "cholesterol doesn't matter" myth, it's time for a reality check. In fact, cholesterol in foods does indeed raise blood cholesterol levels, increasing your risk of heart problems. In 2002, the Institute of Medicine carefully laid out the evidence showing that cholesterol you eat—in eggs, cheese, chicken, beef, or anything else—raises your blood cholesterol level.[26] The evidence was solid and unimpeachable.

So what was the Dietary Guidelines committee up to? Well, it turned out that neither the public, nor the media, nor most of the Dietary Guidelines Advisory Committee members themselves realized that cholesterol's attempted image makeover was, for the most part, an industry-orchestrated effort. To try to rehabilitate cholesterol's image, the egg industry stacked the deck on the Dietary Guidelines Advisory Committee as well as it could. It nominated one scientist who was then placed on the committee, paid for the research of another, and wrote out a check for more than $100,000 in research funds to the university that was home to two more committee members. The egg industry also bankrolled most of the recent research on dietary cholesterol's health effects, designing studies in such a way as to try to minimize cholesterol's apparent dangers.

The good news is that, in the end, industry's attempt at a cholesterol whitewash failed. The government rejected the committee's "cholesterol is safe" notion and said that, in fact, people should eat as little cholesterol as possible. Unfortunately, many people remember the headlines suggesting there is no need to worry about cholesterol's dangers.

Feeling Great Again

Marc and Kim love their new lives. They have energy they never had before. They go kayaking in northern Michigan and have the stamina to work out as often as they feel like it. And since Marc's erectile dysfunction disappeared, they are burning more calories in the bedroom, too. Being active is a joy, not a chore.

They decided to share what they have found. They now teach classes on nutrition and health and bring in doctors, chefs, and other guest lecturers to teach at regular meetings for anyone and everyone who would like to improve their eating habits. Marc and Kim are frequently featured in local news stories, and they set up a fun and informative website, called Chickpea and Bean (ChickpeaAndBean.com) to share recipes, news, and information about upcoming events.

By now, it is clear that getting cheese out of your diet can really boost your health. And food choices raise other issues, too, including their effects on animals and on the environment, as we will see in the next chapter.

CHAPTER 7

What the Animals Go Through

It was a beautiful summer day in Amagansett—a small town on Long Island where the rich go to play. My organization, the Physicians Committee for Responsible Medicine, was having a fund-raiser at a beautiful seaside home and, in honor of the occasion, Michael Schwarz unveiled his brand new *Treeline* cheese.

Michael is an intellectual property attorney who had taken on a new challenge. For reasons I will describe in a moment, he had launched a company producing nondairy cheeses that aimed to rival the traditional varieties. After months of testing and perfecting, it was time for a tasting.

Michael opened up an aged cheese seasoned with black pepper, and the guests, including actor Alec Baldwin, jumped in to give it a try. At first, they wondered if such a tasty cheese could really be dairy-free. It most certainly was. This new cheese was delicious, and it was made without so much as a drop of milk.

I was too busy talking with our guests to taste anything. But Michael wrapped up a packet for me to sample later on. Driving to the airport late that night, I found it in my pocket, pulled off a chunk, and popped it in my mouth. It was wonderful. Perfect flavor, perfect texture, perfectly seasoned. Before I knew it, I had eaten the entire package.

I am introducing you to Michael because his work brings up a side of cheese that we have not yet touched on. It is not something that cheese mongers want to tell you about. But it is important, and it begins, not in New York or Wisconsin, but in Johannesburg.

Michael's father, Harry Schwarz, immigrated to South Africa as a boy, fleeing Germany with his family as the Nazis came to power. Speaking neither English nor Afrikaans, he was taunted and harassed by the other children. But he was a good student, and he grew up fast. After graduation in 1943, he joined the South African Air Force to fight the Nazis in North Africa, Crete, and Italy.

When World War II ended, Harry returned to his adopted home in South Africa, only to find new troubles brewing. The National Party was in its ascendancy and was pushing for the adoption of apartheid. There had been racially unfair policies previously, but this new system of segregation was far more extreme than anything the country had ever known. To Harry, apartheid was akin to the racial and ethnic prejudices he had seen in Germany and had fought against in the war. Along with other veterans, Harry organized marches in an effort to stop it. They failed. Apartheid was institutionalized in 1948.

Harry went to law school, where he began a lifelong friendship with Nelson Mandela, and later defended one of Mandela's co-defendants in the now-infamous Rivonia Trial. Harry's wife, Annette, shared his ethical convictions. She worked at a labor union at a time when blacks were not allowed to unionize, and her union made it a point to advocate for their rights.

Michael carries bitter memories of the racial divide. He remembers sitting on a bus after a sports match at his all-white high school, when the other children stuck their heads out of the windows to spit on black workers who were walking home. He also felt profoundly disturbed at the way the apartheid system broke up families, forcing parents to leave their children in faraway "homelands" because they were not allowed to bring them to the whites-only areas where they worked—the only option available so they could make enough money to support them. As his school's representative at the Johannesburg Junior City Council at sixteen years of age, he aimed to do what he could to change things. He introduced a charter that held that blacks should be allowed to join the council and that apartheid should end. His proposal was resoundingly defeated, and, when he received his diploma at the end of the year, the other students booed and hissed.

Tumultuous times continued during his university years, as Michael protested against apartheid and pushed for Mandela's release. One day, his father, now an outspoken opposition member of parliament, was approached by the head of the national security police who let him know that he and Michael were being watched.

In 1991, when apartheid finally ended, Harry Schwarz was named the South African ambassador to the U.S.—the first ambassador to have openly opposed apartheid. He had steadfastly refused to be an ambassador representing only South Africa's five million whites, saying, "I've made it clear that I want to be ambassador for thirty-seven million people."

The ethical grounding that Michael had had since childhood affected many aspects of his life, including his food choices. At age twenty-seven, he was struck by the fate of animals on farms and in slaughterhouses. People do not need to eat meat, he reasoned. Why put animals through a bleak existence for a burger or lamb chop?

Dairy cows, however, were not on his ethical radar, at least not yet. Quite the reverse. He had fond memories of the Welsh rarebit and grilled cheese sandwiches his mother made when he came home from school. And when his father returned from business trips in Europe, he always brought a package of delicious French cheese that the family enjoyed together. He appreciated the taste of Gorgonzola on bread with jam or honey and grated Parmesan on pasta or straight out of the pack. Later on, Michael traveled to France and Italy for his legal work and sampled the local cheeses—fontina, Camembert, and everything else.

Where Milk Comes From

When Michael was about forty, he learned some disturbing things.

To state the obvious, cows produce milk to nourish their babies. And just as a nursing mother produces enough milk for her baby—not enough to feed the entire neighborhood—a cow normally produces the milk her calf needs and not a lot extra for making cheese and ice cream.

But a dairy farm can't make money that way. So dairy producers do several things. First, they impregnate the cows annually and take the calves away so the dairy can take *all* the milk. Second, through breeding and sometimes using pharmaceuticals, they push cows to produce more milk. Third, when the cows don't earn their keep, they become hamburger and are replaced by younger cows who begin the cycle of impregnation and lactation.

Let's take a closer look at what Michael was concerned about, starting with a trip to northwest Indiana.

Fair Oaks Farms is a massive dairy operation. But it is more than that. It is also a slick showcase for the industry. Welcoming visitors with tours, elaborate displays, a restaurant, and play areas for children, it gives a Disney-like feel to the milk-production process.

On the drive into Fair Oaks Farms, we answer the question we posed back in Chapter 1—why are there so few cows in the Midwestern countryside? It's because they are here, indoors—32,000 of them.

Hop on the bus and take the tour. The Fair Oaks Farms guide will proudly show you the "free-stall barns" where some cows sit "freely"—meaning they are fenced in small indoor groups, rather than individual stalls.

Among Fair Oaks' displays is a video that shows where babies come from. It starts with artificial insemination. No, cows do not choose their mates. In the highly mechanized breeding process of a dairy operation, every aspect of reproduction is controlled by the farm staff, and the video shows the procedure in detail.

The farm will not let you go to watch the process in person. But it did give an up-close look to Mike Rowe for his Discovery Channel program *Dirty Jobs*. For eight seasons, the program covered all manner of difficult and undesirable jobs, and this one was among the most eye-opening.

Mike Rowe first introduces us to Joe, who provides bull semen. Yes, surprising as it sounds, there really are people like Joe who have dedicated their lives to bull semen. Joe knows his bulls, and he selects his samples based on the cows' physical characteristics. A short cow will get semen from a tall bull, for example, aiming to produce a medium-sized calf that the dairy can use. He can

even choose sperm samples that carry either X chromosomes or
Y chromosomes, producing female and male calves, respectively.

For the insemination itself, Tony arrives. Tony has the selected
semen samples in huge containers in the back of his truck. One
by one, he defrosts them and loads them into an insemination
gun that looks like a long knitting needle. On Tony's left arm is a
long plastic sleeve covered with feces from the inseminations he
has just finished.

The cows are lined up next to each other like customers
at bank teller windows. And now we find out where the feces
came from. Tony selects a cow and shoves his left arm deeply
into the cow's rectum. Through the rectal wall, he feels for the
uterus. With his right hand, he grabs the tail of the neighboring
cow and uses it to sponge away the manure that is dribbling
down the cow's backside. He then takes the insemination gun
in hand and pushes it into the cow's vagina and through the

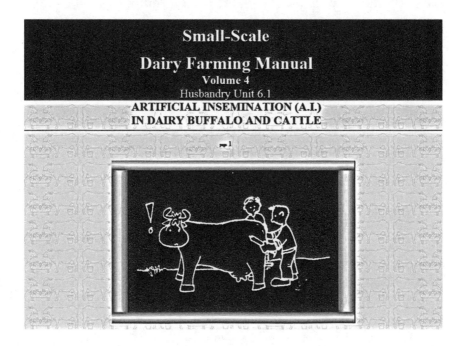

Small-Scale

Dairy Farming Manual
Volume 4
Husbandry Unit 6.1
ARTIFICIAL INSEMINATION (A.I.)
IN DAIRY BUFFALO AND CATTLE

cervix to inject the semen. Mission accomplished, he removes the gun, pulls out his arm, shakes off the extra feces, and writes the date on the cow's flank with a huge marker. Mike tries to follow suit—after all, that's the point of the show—but he repeatedly balks at the repugnant task before finally doing his best to succeed at the job.

If you would like the details, the Food and Agriculture Organization of the United Nations shows the process in its *Small-Scale Dairy Farming Manual*,[1] illustrating it with simple cartoons. The semen is collected from a bull using an "artificial vagina" and is introduced to the cow with the procedure we saw at Fair Oaks Farms.

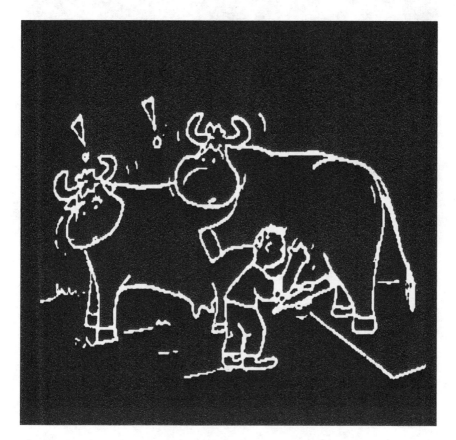

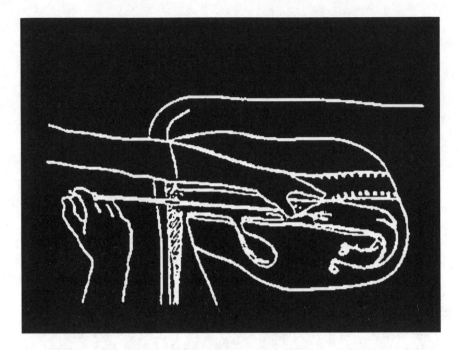

In another part of the farm, the cows who had been impregnated nine months earlier are now giving birth. One is lying down and groaning. We see a tiny hoof appear, then another, and then the baby's head. Soon the calf is born. The mother licks her infant, who takes his first breaths of air and looks around at the strange new world. Calves are born here all day every day, and some of the birthing cows are put on display in a glass enclosure inside an amphitheater for the public to watch.

What's Missing in This Picture?

On *Dirty Jobs*, Mike Rowe shows up with a newborn calf in a wheelbarrow. She struggles to stand up and falls down clumsily. Conspicuously absent is her mother. In fact, there are no mothers in sight anywhere. There are only confused-looking newborn calves.

"After the mothers lick them clean," Mike says, "the calves are brought here to the 'maternity ward' where they have twenty-four hours to get themselves acclimated to life." The calf will be placed in an individual hutch and, a day or two later, she will be sent outside where she will grow for thirteen months, after which she will be impregnated by Tony or one of the other farmhands, just as her mother was.

The Fair Oaks tour guide will show the calves to you. Driving along a roadway, here they are. They are not with their mothers. They are in individual hutches in a long row, one after the other.

What the Fair Oaks tour guide did not describe and what *Dirty Jobs* did not show was the reaction of the mothers as their calves are taken away. Cows do not give up their calves willingly. As farmers load them up, their mothers cry out and vainly try to follow until being turned back. The strength of the mother-infant bond is obvious as the cows call out inconsolably.

Mothers' Laments

On October 23, 2013, the *Daily News* of Newburyport, Massachusetts, reported this story:[2]

> NEWBURY—Strange noises coming from High Road near Sunshine Dairy Farm Monday night and into yesterday morning prompted local police to alert residents that there's nothing spooky or scary going on.
>
> According to Newbury police sergeant Patty Fisher, the noises are coming from mother cows who are lamenting the separation from their calves.
>
> "It happens every year at the same time," she said.

The news story was headlined "Strange Noises Turn Out to Be Cows Missing Their Calves."

(continued)

William Shakespeare used similar words four centuries earlier, in Part 2 of *Henry VI*:

> Thou never didst them wrong, nor no man wrong;
> And as the butcher takes away the calf
> And binds the wretch, and beats it when it strays,
> Bearing it to the bloody slaughter-house,
> Even so remorseless have they borne him hence;
> And as the dam runs lowing up and down,
> Looking the way her harmless young one went,
> And can do nought but wail her darling's loss…

The female calf in Mike Rowe's wheelbarrow will end up as
a part of the dairy herd. Male calves have a different fate. For
eighteen to twenty weeks, they will be fed a milk replacer made
of whey or soy protein, and will then be trucked to a slaughter-
house, hung up by one of their rear legs, and have their throats
slit. The calf's stomach can be preserved for its rennet; the calf
would have used it to digest his mother's milk, had he had the
chance to drink it.

For a female, things are just getting started. Her horns are
removed, often without anesthesia, through processes called
dehorning or *disbudding* (the removal of the horn's growth ring
with a knife or cautery), unless she is lucky enough to have
been bred to have no horns.

She will be impregnated annually, and each calf will be
taken away. Around four years of age, her flagging milk production will not justify the cost of feed, and she will be loaded
onto a truck and sent to slaughter, just like the male calves she
produced.

Many people who object to the slaughter of cows or other
animals imagine that dairy cows are not killed. But, of course,
they are killed, too. They must first go through a few cycles of

impregnation, birth, loss of their calves, and milk production, and then they are slaughtered for their meat and leather.

Milk and Manure

Back in Indiana, we now arrive at the milking process itself. If you imagined a farmer sitting on a stool with a bucket and a good grip, well, this is not what you imagined. A long manure-covered walkway leads to a gigantic rotary device. It is an enormous turntable capable of carrying seventy-two cows at a time. Each cow steps into her slot.

Manure is everywhere—underfoot, on the cows' legs, and on the workers' hands and clothing. To prevent it from sticking to the downy hair on the cows' udders, a veterinarian aims a small flame-thrower over the udder to singe the hair. As the cow kicks, the men discuss whether or not the flames are painful.

Then the milking machine is attached, and in eight and a half minutes, the turntable carries the cow in a circle, and the process is done. Each cow is milked three times a day—five hundred per hour—all day and all night.

For every gallon of milk, a typical cow also produces about two gallons of manure (that is about eight gallons of milk and fifteen gallons of manure each day). If you asked, "Does manure get into the milk?" the more appropriate question might be, "*How much* gets into the milk?" The farm collects 350,000 gallons of milk daily, and lots and lots and lots of manure.

Manure management is a challenge for the milk industry, so much so that there is a magazine devoted to it, entitled, appropriately enough, *Manure Manager.* And the greatest minds in the manure world get together at the North American Manure Expo to discuss how to deal with it and, when possible, score some cash by turning feces into methane gas.

No Kidding

Goats are smaller than cows, and you might think they would be treated a bit better. But you would be disappointed. Like cows, goats produce milk for their offspring, not for any other purpose. So producing cheese means impregnating the females, taking away the kids, and eventually killing more or less all of them.

Goats are typically impregnated annually, like cows. Most of the kids have to go, if the dairy is going to keep the milk for sale—although it can add some of the females to the dairy herd and can raise some of the males for meat.

To prevent the goats from hurting the farm personnel or each other, dairy farmers remove the horns. They can actually burn away the horn buds with an electric iron before the horns have grown. If that sounds painful—and it is—it only gets worse when the horns have started to grow. They are then cut off by dehorning. Have a look at this advice from *Storey's Guide to Raising Dairy Goats*, from Storey Publishing:[3]

> Dehorning can be quite painful and even dangerous to the goat, and so upsetting to the surgeon that even many trained veterinarians won't do it, and those who do it once won't repeat the performance. (p. 114)
>
> Each horn must be removed close to the skull, and a thin slice of the skull taken with it, or the horn will grow back. There will be a great deal of blood, the decidedly unpleasant view into the sinus cavities of the goat, the real risk of having to deal with infection, and the obvious difficulty of controlling an adult animal. (p. 117)

If you're going to raise them for meat, you'll want to castrate the males in order to avoid having "buck odor" in the meat.

The *Guide* says that "until they are about one month old, bucks can be surgically castrated without anesthesia"—reminiscent of the days when pediatric surgeons thought that babies had such immature nervous systems that they did not feel pain. They were clearly and tragically wrong.

Wait a minute! I just wanted some cheese. Who said anything about ripping out their horns, cutting off their testicles, and raising goats for meat? Well, the fact is, *essentially all dairy goats are eventually slaughtered for meat, just like dairy cows.* The *Guide* tells us:

> Meat is an important by-product of dairying. Over the years any farm will average 50 percent buck kids. Not one in a hundred can be kept, profitably, as a herd sire. While there is a limited demand for wethers (castrated males) as pets in some areas, it is more merciful in most cases to butcher them for meat.
>
> In addition to unwanted males, any dairy operation will have cull or aged does that simply are not paying their way... Culling is a fact of life...Butchering is never a pleasant task, and it's normal to have qualms about eating an animal you raised yourself. (p. 218)

Yes, the *Guide* says, "let's face it, many goat raisers can't even think of butchering and eating kids. But if your little herd doubles or triples in size every year, something has to give."(p. 161)

Taking a Stand

All of this would be troubling to anyone. And for Michael Schwarz, whose family had long fought against the abuse and exploitation of human beings—particularly the forced separation of parents from their children to provide cheap labor—it was hard to ignore the parallel experience in animals.

"I learned that dairy cows are killed and that their calves are killed, too—and that before death they live lives of misery," he said. "Think about taking an animal, forcing her to have a baby, taking her baby away, and stealing her milk. That is bullying. The most powerful bond we know of is the bond between mother and child, and we break it in order to make 'comfort foods' for ourselves."

For a while, Michael bought organic cheese, trying to persuade himself that the animals must have been treated better. "Soon, I realized this was simply not true. It was a myth I wanted to believe to justify my taste for Gorgonzola. When I realized that, I had to stop buying it."

Michael did better than that. He launched a nondairy cheese company that made it easy for everyone to enjoy a food product that is both delicious and ethically produced. In Chapter 10, I'll show you how he did it.

The Environment

It's not just the animals who have a rough time. The environment does, too—in many ways. A full description of the effects of food choices on the environment could easily fill this entire book. But let me share just a few key points:

Water: There are roughly 100 million cows in North America, and each one is as big as a sofa. If you could put all the humans in North America on one side of a balance and all the cows on the other side, the cows would massively outweigh us. And if you then think about what it takes to feed the human population, it takes far more than that to feed cows. Cows eat a huge amount of food.

Without a steady supply of feed grain, dairies and slaughterhouses would grind to a halt. Millions of acres are devoted to planting corn, soybeans, and other feed crops, not for human consumption, but to feed animals. And those crops need water—more, in fact, than any other human activity. If water does not come from the sky, it has to come from irrigation. Producing cheese means a huge drain of water to irrigate feed crops so that cows produce the milk that is then concentrated in cheese.

Pollution: Feed crops also require fertilizer, and some of the nitrogen and phosphorus in fertilizer dribbles into rivers and streams, disturbing the ecosystem. It stimulates algae overgrowth, which, in turn, uses up oxygen from the water. Without oxygen, fish die. Farmers and the environmental protection groups are well aware of it. But they have not figured out a way to dump countless tons of fertilizers on the land without some of it ending up in waterways.

In the Gulf of Mexico, directly below Texas and Louisiana, is an 8,000-square-mile dead zone, caused by the fertilizer runoff from the Mississippi River. It is there thanks to the farms all along the Mississippi and the many rivers running into it.

If people ate plants directly, instead of the products of animals raised on feed crops, there would be much less need for irrigation and fertilizer, and the Gulf dead zone would likely recover.

Climate change: You have one stomach. Cows have four, and they digest food very differently. Being ruminants, they belch methane gas, which happens to be a potent greenhouse gas. It traps heat, and is much more powerful in this regard than carbon dioxide. If there were simply a cow here and a cow there, this would not matter. But with 100 million cows, it is a major contributor to global climate change. So while governments debate about smokestack emissions and environmental groups complain that little is being done, the fact is that we can tackle the biggest part of climate change simply by changing our eating habits.

Fixing It

A great many people have turned away from meat-eating because of the grotesque cruelty involved. But dairying can claim no ethical advantage. The industry relies on impregnating animals, separating them from their infants, pushing them to produce as much milk as drugs and biology can manage, and killing them as soon as it no longer pays to keep them alive.

The dairy industry and the feed-crop production that it requires are massively environmentally unfriendly. And everything that goes into making milk is, of course, multiplied by ten to make that concentrated product called cheese. With all of these revelations, cheese has a distinctly unpleasant odor about it.

Even though many of the details in this chapter may be new to you, you no doubt already realized that animals on farms were not exactly having a picnic. Other people recognize that, too. So why are we so slow to change? If we understand that our eating habits are killing a million animals *every hour* and are steadily damaging the Earth itself, why are we not collectively throwing our cheese packages and steak knives in the trash and vowing to make a better world?

The reason is simple: Logic plays only a very small role in human behavior. And I would argue that that is, for the most part, a good thing. Here is what I mean: If a sheep were to think logically about whether that sound in the distance really is a wolf, and she were to try to calculate the time it might take for the wolf to attack and assess the probability that other wolves might be nearby, that unfortunate sheep would be killed. Instead, sheep run. If the herd is going, each individual sheep is heading out, too.

Something similar is true of chimpanzees. In her research in Tanzania, Jane Goodall observed that, if an infant chimpanzee happens to pick a berry or blossom that the group does not eat, his mother or aunt is likely to stop him before he can put it into his mouth. There is safety in sticking with the group.

Humans are much the same. We don't base our food choices on ethics or logic, for the most part. We eat more or less the way our parents or friends eat, and we take comfort in not deviating too far from the pack. That is understandable. Smokers had the same false sense of safety until their friends started to get nervous and began to quit smoking.

More and more people are making the same choice that Michael did, saying that they simply cannot be part of a cruel system any longer. And when they make changes in order to be more ethical, they get the added health advantages as a bonus.

Meanwhile, the dairy industry is working hard to keep notions like these from entering your mind. In the next chapter, we will see the surprising lengths it goes to to protect its market.

CHAPTER 8

The Industry Behind the Addiction

Wisconsin Avenue. It's a good address for a group taking on the cheese industry.

In their offices at the Physicians Committee for Responsible Medicine's headquarters in Washington, DC, Mark Kennedy and Mindy Kursban were combing through government records like bloodhounds tracking a criminal. The Physicians Committee is the organization I founded in 1985 to promote better nutrition, better health, and better research. Mindy and Mark are attorneys. Mindy was educated at Emory University, Mark at Washington and Lee.

Using the Freedom of Information Act, they had unearthed a stack of contracts between the government and fast-food chains to push cheese, grants to researchers aiming to make dairy products look healthy, and advertising schemes aimed at boosting cheese sales. In this chapter, I'll share what they found. If you imagined that food industry giants have your best interests at heart, you will find some new things to think about.

Triggering Cheese Craving

Exhibit A: The Cheese Forum.

Among the documents these legal sleuths uncovered was a presentation, dated December 5, 2000, at what was called a "Cheese Forum." Dick Cooper, the vice president of cheese marketing for Dairy Management Inc., was about to unveil a new plan to boost cheese sales across America. He took to the podium. "What do we want our marketing program to do?" he asked the audience of industry execs.

"Hmmm. Good question," the audience was no doubt thinking. "How are we going to promote cheese? Ask convenience stores to put cheese displays near the registers? Find a celebrity to pose with a wheel of Cheddar? Give away samples on street corners?"

No, those are small-time ideas. The cheese industry is far more creative than that. And Dick Cooper gave the answer: "Trig-

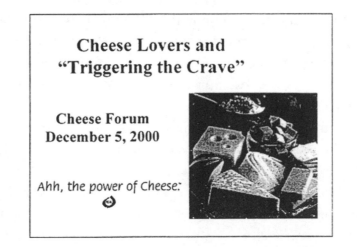

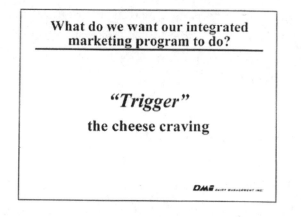

ger the cheese craving." The idea was not to make cheese sound tasty or to show how practical it can be in a sandwich. The plan was to work inside consumers' heads—and *get America hooked.*

Cooper made his case. Customers can be divided into two categories, he said. "Enhancers" are people who sprinkle a little mozzarella on a salad or grind some Parmesan on pasta. Forget them; they are not worth targeting. The group to go after was labeled "cravers"—people who open the refrigerator door, break off a chunk of cheese, and stuff it in their mouths as is. Cravers *love* cheese, and, with a little prompting, they will double or triple their cheese intake.

So, how do you trigger food cravings? Just ask anyone who ever smelled fresh popcorn walking into a movie theater, anyone who ever walked past a bakery, or any baseball fan who ever smelled stadium hot dogs. If you were in these situations, you weren't necessarily thinking about these foods at first, but all of a sudden they leapt into your world and you *had* to have them. So, industry's trick is to use suggestions—subtle or not—that bring the product to mind as often as possible, and then make sure that the product is widely available so that your craving leads to a purchase. Cravings can be triggered, and people aiming to push food products know it.

What was most surprising was that this marketing program—designed to fuel food addiction—was not launched by Kraft, Sargento, or the cheese makers of Normandy. It was a program of the U.S. government.

Your Government at Work

Here's how it works: The U.S. government collects money from dairy producers and hands it over to an outfit called Dairy Management Inc. (DMI). Right now, the amount totals about $140 million a year, and DMI uses it to push cheese and other dairy products.

DMI's story actually starts a century ago. In 1915, a foot-and-mouth disease outbreak threatened the image of the dairy industry, and the National Dairy Council was formed for damage control. Over the years, industry programs promoting milk and other dairy products have grown, and in 1983, the government took on a new role for the industry. The Dairy and Tobacco Adjustment Act created a federal board for dairy promotions, and eventually the government consolidated these programs under DMI.

You might be asking why the government is involved in cheese marketing at all. After all, it doesn't provide marketing services for shoes, computers, make-up, or plumbing supplies. Why cheese? The answer has nothing to do with health. It has to do with money and politics.

As we've seen, DMI's plan was, in essence, to make cheese inescapable—the equivalent of having popcorn not just in theaters, but just about everywhere. But how to do that? If you guessed "blow cheesy smells through air vents," "ask the president to wear a cheese hat during the State of the Union address," or "change the song lyrics from 'amber waves of grain' to 'ample waves of Colby and American process cheese spread,'" you'd be wrong. DMI realized that the way to reach into every city and town in America was through fast-food chains. A single corporate decision can affect what tens of millions of people eat every day.

So DMI contracted with Wendy's to push a Cheddar-Lover's Bacon Cheeseburger. During the promotional period, Wendy's

---

O'Connell, Norton & Partners

O'Connell, Norton & Partners
625 North Michigan Avenue
Chicago, IL 60611-3110
Tel: 312-988-3500
Fax: 312-988-3576

Mr. Derek Correia
Director, Product Marketing   May 11, 2000
Burger King
17777 Old Cutler Road
Miami, Florida 33157

Re: Agreement between Dairy Management Inc. and Burger King Corp.

Dear Derek:

This Letter Agreement ("Agreement"), made on this the 3rd day of March, 2000, is by and between O'Connell, Norton & Partners, a division of Bozell Group ("Agency"), as agent for its client, Dairy Management Inc. ("DMI") and Burger King Corp. ("Company") for the purpose of carrying out the activities described below. In consideration of the mutual covenants and agreements contained herein, the parties agree as follows:

1. **Project Description.**

   A. Menu Concept Development. DMI and Agency will conduct two idea sessions (one for the entry segment and one for the indulgent segment) to develop new menu concepts and to make recommendations for new menu concepts featuring cheese for consideration by Company (hereafter "Menu Concept Development" research). DMI and Agency will provide written descriptions of up to 25 new items from each session for Company consideration and further testing (qualitative and quantitative). Participants in each Menu Concept Development may include chefs, a consumer specialist, a culinary expert, a food scientist as well as consumers. DMI agrees to fund this Menu Concept Development research.

sold 2.25 million pounds of cheese. DMI worked with Sub-way to market Chicken Cordon Bleu and Honey Pepper Melt sandwiches. It contracted with Pizza Hut to unveil the Ultimate Cheese Pizza with an entire pound of cheese in a single serving. DMI worked with Burger King, Taco Bell, and all the other fast-food chains to trigger cheese craving in the same way that movies, bakeries, and baseball parks—intentionally or not—promote cravings of their own.

Under contract with DMI, the chains put more cheese items on the menu, put cheese slogans on the cashiers' hats, and did their best to make customers choose cheese instead of salad. You might not have been thinking about cheese when you walked through the restaurant door, but DMI aimed to make it inescapable. It's everywhere.

What!? The government is intentionally promoting *cheese craving*? The same government that is supposedly interested in our health—it's trying to make us *crave cheese*? You bet. No matter how fattening and cholesterol-laden cheese may be, by law, the government has to promote it, thanks to the relentless lobbying of the powerful dairy industry that led to the creation of a broad range of federal dairy-promotion programs. And it has worked. Cheese sales have climbed year after year.

At a meeting in Phoenix in 2013, DMI CEO Tom Gallagher listed the program's successes.[1] Since 2009, DMI's pizza partnerships had turned ten billion extra pounds of milk into cheese for pizza. DMI provided staff to McDonald's headquarters to build the company's expertise and sales. Gallagher projected that its partnership with Taco Bell alone would sell the cheese equivalent of 1.7 billion pounds of milk in 2013, and two billion more in 2014. And the program worked overseas, too. Contracts with Domino's, Pizza Hut, and Papa John's moved more than 100 million pounds of cheese in Pacific Rim countries.

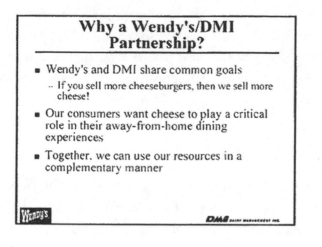

Propping Up Sales

If it surprises you that the cheese industry has managed to insinuate its way into the government, this is just the beginning. The industry-government partnership also has a special way of targeting children. When cheese prices fall, the government buys cheese to boost farm income. Similarly, when beef prices fall, the government buys beef. Suddenly, children in schools find more cheeseburgers in their lunch lines. In fiscal year 2015, the government's Agricultural Marketing Service bought more than 160 million pounds of cheese, at a cost of nearly $300 million.

As I drafted this chapter, I checked the menu for the District of Columbia Public Schools. And, yes, cheese was all over it. There was pizza, "hand crafted in our kitchen on whole grain crusts." There was a Steak and Cheese Sub, a Cheese and Yogurt Platter, a Toasted Two Cheese Sandwich, and cheeseburgers. And just in case kids had not had enough cheese already, they would find shredded Cheddar at the salad bar.

So, does this mean that all the while that Michelle Obama was campaigning against childhood obesity, the USDA was working to push cheese sales? That is exactly what it means, and I don't need to tell you who won. The government programs that push cheese were there long before Mrs. Obama's *Let's Move* campaign was launched and, if nothing changes, will be there well into the future.

Money and Politics

This does not mean the food industry is indifferent to health. Quite the opposite. The industry is keenly interested in health—or, more specifically, what you *believe* to be healthy.

Every five years, the U.S. government revises the Dietary Guidelines for Americans. These guidelines are the blueprint for all nutrition programs in the U.S., and a model for many other countries, as well. The revision is led by a committee appointed by the USDA and the Department of Health and Human Services.

The committee hearings are a spectacle to behold. The committee members take their seats on a stage in a large auditorium. In front of them, a microphone is plugged in, and one by one, speakers step up to make a three-minute pitch. Representatives from the National Dairy Council, the National Cattlemen's Beef Association, the Sugar Association, the Salt Institute, the Chocolate Council, the liquor industry, and everyone else with something to sell tell the committee members why their products should be part of the American diet. The committee then weighs the testimony and whatever other evidence it can gather and issues its report.

As the guidelines were being revised for the year 2000, Mindy Kursban noticed something peculiar. Digging into the résumés of the Dietary Guidelines Advisory Committee members, she found that one had been given a $42,000 grant from

DMI, along with fellowships from Kraft, the maker of Velveeta and other cheese products. Another committee member had received a half-million-dollar grant from a company making dairy-based products. A third had received grant payments from the National Dairy Promotion and Research Board and the National Live Stock and Meat Board. The committee chair had been a paid consultant with the National Dairy Council and Dannon—the yogurt company—and had also been paid more than $10,000 by Nestlé Switzerland, a maker of ice cream and other milk products. Of the eleven committee members, six had financial ties to the dairy, meat, or egg industry.

Financial ties are not necessarily off limits for government panels. After all, if the Pentagon is buying new aircraft, it might want advice from Boeing, Lockheed Martin, Embraer, and whomever else might have detailed knowledge and something to say. But if most of the panel members were from one manufacturer, it would obviously not be good. So the government has a law—called the Federal Advisory Committee Act—that requires balance, and bars inappropriate special interest influence.

So, on behalf of the Physicians Committee, Mindy filed suit in the United States District Court for the District of Columbia. We did not have the funding, legal staff, or clout that industry and government have. But it helps when you are right. On September 30, 2000, U.S. District Judge James Robertson laid down his decision. We won our case. The government had violated the law, he ruled, and had to clean up its act.

Ever since, the process has gotten better. Yes, the food industry reps still stand up to the microphone every five years to plead their case to the Dietary Guidelines Advisory Committee, and they work behind the scenes to influence committee members. But the government panel is more careful than in the past, and industries are finding it harder and harder to fight the mountain of research showing the risks of meat and dairy products and the value of truly healthful foods.

Truth and Advertising

On May 3, 2007, the U.S. government did something it practically never does. It stood up to the dairy industry.

Two years earlier, Mindy and Mark had gone to the Federal Trade Commission with dairy advertisements in hand. The dairy industry was making an extraordinary claim, that dairy products promote weight loss.

"Wow!" you might be thinking. "That's a good one. Milk fattens calves, and now it is going to make me slim!"

The notion came from Dr. Michael Zemel, a researcher at the University of Tennessee. Dr. Zemel conducted experiments in mice, which, he said, showed that boosting calcium intake could accelerate weight loss. He then reported the same result in people. Overweight individuals who cut calories seemed to lose more weight when dairy products were part of their low-calorie diets, compared with just cutting calories alone.

Based on his research, the dairy industry advertising machinery started humming. An ad from Kraft showed a sweaty block of cheese emblazoned with the words "Burn More Fat." The ad copy said, "Good News. Recent studies show including the recommended amount of CALCIUM from dairy products like KRAFT Cheese, in a reduced-calorie diet, may help you **burn more fat** than cutting calories alone." Another, for Kraft Singles, made the same claim. Dr. Phil McGraw appeared in a dairy ad, sporting a milk mustache, with the title "Get real. About losing weight." Milk, cheese, calcium—yes, they are going to slim

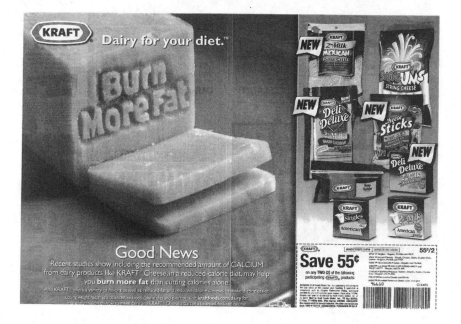

you right down. The weight-loss claim was trumpeted in *People* magazine, *Good Morning America*, and endless other outlets.

But a closer look showed problems. In Dr. Zemel's 2004 article in the journal *Obesity Research*,[2] he disclosed that his research had been paid for by the National Dairy Council. And the study was small—ten people in a control group, and eleven each in a high-calcium and a high-dairy group. Another Zemel study, reaching the same conclusion the following year, was funded by General Mills and was similarly small.[3] Moreover, it turned out that Zemel had patented his dairy–weight loss plan, and had a book to sell, too. It all smelled like money, not science.

Most problematic was that other researchers had been unable to replicate his findings. Researchers from the University of British Columbia had compiled the data in a review published in the *Journal of Nutrition*. Nine studies had looked at experiments to

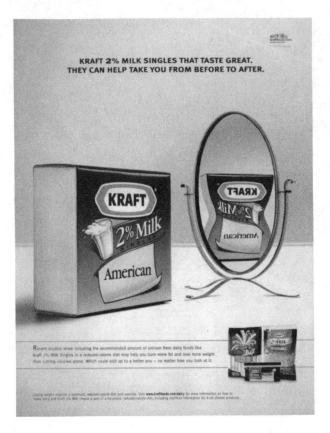

see the effect of dairy products on body weight. None showed any benefit.[4] Drink all the milk you want, they found—it will not help you lose weight.

Our lawyers went to work. First, we asked the Federal Trade Commission to investigate. And to its credit, it did. In the meantime, Kraft's sweaty cheese block had to go. We filed suit against the company, calling on it to stop claiming that cheese or any other dairy product would cause weight loss. Kraft quickly let us know that it would not run the ads any further. And two years later, the Federal Trade Commission pulled the plug on the dairy–weight loss claims altogether.

In the aftermath, our team took one more look at the evidence. And indeed, it does not support any notion that dairy products help you lose weight. We eventually found forty-nine research studies testing the effect of dairy products or of calcium alone, with or without calorie-cutting, and found that the notion that dairy products promote weight loss is clearly a myth.[5] As we saw in Chapter 2, cheese can easily do the opposite. It helps you pack on the pounds.

So, What about All Those Other Claims?

The dairy–weight loss controversy showed a troubling side of the industry. It was dishonest. It was surprisingly eager to make health claims that did not even pass the sniff test. If the weight-loss claim is not real, it makes you wonder, what about all those other claims, like "milk builds strong bones"? That notion has been embedded in our memories since our grade school days and is right up there with Santa Claus and the Easter Bunny in popularity. Could that be on shaky scientific ground, too? Or what about the idea that older women should drink milk to protect against bone breaks? That is a common idea, but what does the science look like?

At Penn State University, researchers launched the Penn State Young Women's Health Study, including eighty adolescent girls who participated for ten years, from age twelve to twenty-two.[6] The researchers followed their diets and exercise patterns. Along the way, they carefully examined their bone strength and integrity.

Their calcium intake covered a wide range. Some got as little as 500 milligrams per day, while others got much more—as much as 1,900 milligrams a day. But it turned out that it did not matter. Variations in calcium intake from milk, cheese, or anything else did not affect their bones. Milk did not make their bones stronger, more resilient, or less likely to break. What did matter was exercise. Those children who exercised more had better bone integrity.

It turns out that, although the body does need some calcium, it does not need an especially large amount of it. The government has been pushing calcium—as much as 1,300 milligrams per day for teenagers. But studies show that, once you are getting about 600 milligrams per day, there is no benefit from going higher. Also, calcium does not have to come from dairy products. It is found in a wide range of much more healthful foods. Beans and green vegetables are at the top of the list (and deserve a big place in everyone's diet), and many other foods contain calcium, too. In addition, dairy products don't "build strong bones." So long as growing children are getting good nutrition, those who skip dairy products have just as good bone development as other kids.[7]

At the other end of the age spectrum, older women—especially older white women—are often told that, because they are at risk for osteoporosis and hip fracture, they should drink milk. The idea is that milk's calcium will shore up their bone strength. Harvard University researchers put the notion to the test in the Nurses' Health Study. Following 72,337 women over an eighteen-year period, the study found that those who drank milk every day had no protection at all from hip fractures.[8]

Well, maybe the women who weren't drinking milk were taking calcium pills, and so milk's benefits were harder to see in the comparison. But that was not the case either. Zeroing in on women who never used calcium supplements, those who drank at least a glass and a half of milk daily actually had slightly *more* bone breaks than those who avoided milk—about 10 percent more. The added fracture risk could have been due to chance, but it was clear that milk was not helping at all.

But maybe old age is too late. Maybe what counts is how much milk you drink when you're young, so you build up your bone strength. That's the idea the dairy industry has pushed. So the Harvard team looked at that, too. It turned out that, among women, milk consumption during adolescence had no effect at all on women's hip fracture risk in older age. The researchers also looked at men. In a large group of men participating in the Health Professionals Follow-Up Study, there was an effect of milk, but it was exactly the opposite of what milk producers would have wanted. Milk-drinking during the teenage years was associated with more—not fewer—bone breaks in later life. Every additional glass of milk consumed per day during adolescence was associated with a 9 percent *increase* in hip fractures in later life.[9]

None of this means that you do not need calcium. You do. But you do not need enormous amounts of it, and you don't need calcium from milk at all. The "milk builds strong bones" idea has been promoted for commercial reasons and has been memorized by parents and children over the generations. But, like the "milk causes weight loss" claim, it is a myth.

Personally, I have found it disturbing that some of the nutritional lessons that have been pounded into our heads since childhood—and that we have accepted as fact—are nothing more than industry marketing schemes. It is also disturbing that the industry is still actively promoting shaky ideas in schools and on television in order to push its products. These notions endure, and they displace helpful information about what really can strengthen bones and promote good health. There is another striking dairy claim that comes from a company in Hagerstown, Maryland. The company makes chocolate milk that is advertised as a sports recovery drink under the name Fifth Quarter Fresh.[10] The University of Maryland tested the product in high school football players.

The lead investigator, Jae Kun Shim, reported stunning results on the University of Maryland website.[11] Kids who drank

Fifth Quarter Fresh did better in cognitive tests. In other words, they were mentally sharper, and that was true, *even if they had suffered football-related concussions.* The university website posted pictures of the magic drink and an endorsement from Clayton Wilcox, superintendent of Washington County Public Schools: "There is nothing more important than protecting our student-athletes. Now that we understand the findings of this study, we are determined to provide Fifth Quarter Fresh to all of our athletes."

However, there is another side to this story, as you have no doubt guessed. The research was paid for through a $100,000 financial arrangement between the dairy company, the university, and the Maryland Industrial Partnerships Program.

As of this writing, the results have not been peer-reviewed or published. However, the university did release a PowerPoint summary of the results, including composite scores for verbal memory, visual memory, processing speed, reaction time, and other measures. As it turns out, none showed any benefit of the milk product that met the usually accepted criterion for statistical significance. In other words, either the product was useless or any benefits observed on one test or another could have been due to random chance.

The notion that athletes should drink chocolate milk has been heavily promoted by the USDA's milk marketing programs, which push chocolate milk at marathons and in paid advertisements featuring athletes posing with chocolate milk containers. So far, there is no sign they are letting up.

Buying Friends

Sometimes, the dairy industry dispenses with trying to convince people of its merits and just buys loyalty with cash.

Take the Academy of Nutrition and Dietetics, for example. Founded as the American Dietetic Association, it changed its name to "AND" in 2012. The organization oversees who can and cannot be a registered dietitian, and, in some states, *only* registered dietitians and very few other professionals are legally allowed to give nutrition counseling. If you're a cheese manufacturer, you would love to have dietitians on your side. They are the ones who give nutrition advice, go on news programs, oversee hospital food services, and do lots of other things that could help or hurt your business.

AND's website includes a page called "Meet Our Sponsors." At the top of the list is the academy's national sponsor, the National Dairy Council. The next level down names its premier sponsor: Abbott Nutrition, which sells dairy-based baby formulas and supplements, such as Ensure.[12]

What? The organization representing America's dietitians is bankrolled by the dairy industry? Actually, the money has piled up pretty fast. AND's 2015 financial report lists $1.2 million in sponsorship contributions, plus $2.1 million in grants and $1.8 million in corporate contributions and sponsorships to the AND Foundation.[13]

AND is not alone. The National Dairy Council pays $10,000 a year to be part of the American Heart Association's Industry Nutrition Advisory Panel. Along with other panel members— Nestlé, Coca-Cola, the Egg Nutrition Center, the Beef Check-off Program, and a handful of other food industry giants—the National Dairy Council is granted special access to AHA's Nutrition Committee—the group that sets AHA policies and weighs in on federal nutrition issues.

The American Academy of Pediatrics is active in nutrition, too, providing guidance on what parents should feed their children. Corporate sponsors are invited to contribute to the AAP's charitable fund. The list includes Dannon, Coca-Cola, and plenty of pharmaceutical manufacturers.[14]

A decade ago, DMI cooked a deal with the American Dietetic Association, the American Academy of Pediatrics, the American Academy of Family Physicians, and the National Medical Association to launch the 3-A-Day program. The idea was that three servings of dairy products daily is the way to fight the "calcium crisis"—which DMI also invented.[15]

These health organizations are well aware that food companies that send them checks are doing so with the sole aim of influencing their nutrition policies: They hope that dietitians will recommend milk instead of green vegetables for calcium, that heart doctors will overlook the load of saturated fat and cholesterol in cheese, and that pediatricians will not worry too much about pudgy pizza-eating children. So these health organizations do maintain policies about conflicts of interest. AND specifically reports, "The Academy's programs, leadership, decisions, policies and positions are not influenced by sponsors." It is fair to say that the sponsors do not believe that and many AND members do not either. A group of dietitians, called Dietitians for Professional Integrity, holds that the country's largest nutrition organization should not be sponsored by food industry giants.[16]

My impression is that industry funding has indeed had a corrupting influence on major health organizations. It continues only because it is so common and longstanding that otherwise good scientists, doctors, and dietitians have simply gotten used to it.

Keeping You in the Dark

Slanted and even dishonest messages, ill-founded advertisements, and buying friends—what else does the food industry do? Two more things that you should know about:

Don't call it cheese. When you buy a wheel from Miyoko's Kitchen—a manufacturer of the creative cashew-based cheeses we will meet in the next chapter—you'll notice that the word "cheese" is nowhere on the package. Ditto for products from Kite Hill and similar producers of nondairy cheeses. That's because in California, the word "cheese" cannot legally be used unless the product is made from dairy milk. The industry hopes that consumers will be less likely to go for a "cultured nut product."

Ag-gag is real. Let's say an undercover investigator finds that cows injected with bovine growth hormone have mastitis—an infected udder—and that milk from a sick cow, along with antibiotics used to treat the condition, might have been sent to a dairy anyway. What if an investigator finds disease-ridden animals or evidence of cruelty on a farm and has video footage to prove it? The agriculture lobby has been working hard to ensure that, if police are called in such an instance, it will be the journalist who is arrested.

In 2013, Amy Meyer was prosecuted under a Utah law for videotaping at Dale T Smith and Sons Meat Packing Company in Draper City, Utah. Amy had seen a cow who appeared to be sick or injured and was being taken away with a tractor, like garbage. She took out her phone and started recording. The manager came out and told her to stop, but Amy refused. Soon, the police arrived. The company was owned by the town mayor, Darrell Smith, and the plan was not to help the cow or clean up the slaughter operation. The plan was to stop any documentation of what went on inside.

The charges against Amy were eventually dropped. But the agriculture lobby continues to push for "ag-gag" laws because it knows the public would be repulsed by the disgusting—and sometimes illegal—activities that go on in these facilities.

Industry Is Alive and Well, Even If You Are Not

The dairy industry is still working hard to keep you hooked and believing the health mythology that it creates. It is busily cooking deals with fast-food chains, buying friends among health experts and health organizations, and lobbying to keep its products prominent in the Dietary Guidelines for Americans. When cheese prices fall, the government still buys it and puts it into schools, regardless of children's real nutritional needs or health challenges. The money the industry has at its disposal has been more than sufficient to dissolve scientific integrity and ethical principles among many organizations that should know better.

But, like Mark and Mindy, a growing number of attorneys, advocates, and health experts have been moved by the health problems, environmental disasters, and animal welfare issues caused by industry and are working hard to expose them. And when members of the public become aware of these problems, there is not enough money in DMI's marketing budget to make them forget.

CHAPTER 9

A Healthy Diet

By now, you are no doubt rethinking whatever love affair you may have had with cheese. Hopefully, you have burned your love letters and resolved to move on.

But a healthy diet means more than chucking out the Velveeta. Breaking a cheese habit is a great step, but you will no doubt want to do more. In this chapter, we will look at what makes up a truly healthful menu and how to make the leap fun and enjoyable.

Feel the Power

Let me first inspire you with a true story about what healthful foods can do.

I would like to introduce you to Patricia, who worked as a Defense Intelligence Agency analyst at the Pentagon. Patricia had struggled with her weight for most of her life. If that had been her only challenge, she would have been lucky. But 2007 brought a diagnosis of diabetes. Her doctor gave her the advice that is familiar to anyone with diabetes—stay away from pasta, potatoes, bread, and rice, because "carbs turn to sugar." But that did not help her diabetes, and even with a combination of oral and injectable medications, her blood sugar levels were barely under control.

The following year, she developed shortness of breath and pain in her jaw and left arm. Her doctors' suspicions proved correct—she had developed severe heart disease. An angiogram showed three completely blocked arteries, another one that was 90 percent blocked, and one 80 percent blocked. Her next stop was the operating room for bypass surgery. After her surgery, the hospital dietitian prescribed a Mediterranean diet. But within three months, her chest pain returned, necessitating more medications. She was now taking two shots and thirteen pills a day.

In 2010, a friend recommended a book I had written about diabetes, which had been inspired by our team's series of research studies, including a major study funded by the National Institutes of Health. Instead of limiting carbs and cutting calories, we took a completely different approach. We threw out animal products, removed all added oils, and focused on an entirely plant-based diet.

As we saw in Chapter 6, type 2 diabetes starts as insulin resistance. That means that insulin, which is supposed to escort glucose into muscle and liver cells, no longer works properly. The reason, it turns out, is fat. That is, microscopic fat droplets building up inside the muscle and liver cells interfere with insulin's action. So instead of limiting calories or avoiding carbohydrate, we should avoid animal products. That means there is no

animal fat in the diet at all. And when oils are kept to a minimum, there is not much of any fat, apart from the traces of fat
that are natural in foods. In theory, these diet changes ought to
make the fat droplets dissipate from the cells. Plus, they ought to
be good for the heart, too, because there is almost no saturated
fat and no cholesterol on your plate.

Patricia gave it a try. "I thought, well, nothing else I had ever
tried to help control my blood sugar had worked before," she
said. "This concept was completely different." And, yes, within
a few months, her diabetes had improved to the point that she
was able to stop her shots and cut her oral diabetes medications
in half.

Unfortunately, junk food eventually lured her back, and her
health suffered a turn for the worse. She regained lost weight,
her diabetes worsened, and her joints started to ache with arthritis. In 2014, she found herself in the Cleveland Clinic for more
heart surgery. She was sent home with eight stents.

That was her wake-up call. This really was a matter of life
and death. No more junk. No more meat, dairy, or grease. And
she transformed her life.

She is now 95 pounds lighter. From two shots and thirteen
pills, she is down to a half pill per day. "My doctor has purged
diabetes from my medical records. I love this way of life and the
power that I have since I finally took control of my body," she
said.

Her husband joined her in her new way of eating. In the process, he lost 38 pounds and his arthritis went away.

But is it difficult? No, it's surprisingly easy. "We never miss
the meat," she said. "One of my favorite simple dinners is a
baked Japanese sweet potato piled high with steamed kale,
pinto beans, chopped red pepper, scallions, and mango with

salsa. Delicious. We also love stir-fried vegetables over brown rice and pasta primavera. And gone are the diabetes, angina, weight issues, sugar cravings, low energy, and arthritis."

We have heard from hundreds of people like Patricia whose lives have been transformed by simple food changes. Let's look at the foods that work this magic.

What's In

The foods that support health come in four groups: vegetables, fruits, whole grains, and legumes. Let's look at each one and the meals they turn into. Then we'll look at what's out.

To keep things simple, the Power Plate, developed by my organization, the Physicians Committee for Responsible Medicine, depicts the foods that support good health.

- **Vegetables:** Vegetables are loaded with vitamins, minerals, and antioxidants, with essentially no "bad fats" or cholesterol. Bring on the green vegetables: broccoli, kale,

The Power Plate

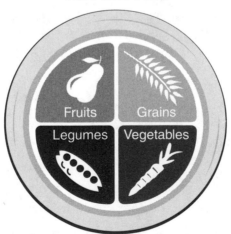

spinach, Brussels sprouts, and all the rest. If you're not yet a vegetable lover, try a spritz of soy sauce, seasoned vinegar, or Bragg liquid aminos. And try the orange vegetables, too—sweet potatoes and carrots, for example. I'd suggest including two or more vegetables at each meal.

- **Legumes:** The legume group includes beans, peas, and lentils—foods that grow in a pod. So that might mean kidney beans, black beans, pinto beans, chickpeas, and all the foods these humble beans turn into, like hummus, tofu, and soy milk. Beans are rich in healthful protein, calcium, iron, and fiber.
- **Whole grains:** Grains are staples in most culinary traditions: rice in Asia, corn in Latin America, wheat in Europe. Many cultures remove the bran coating from grains, turning brown rice into white rice and brown bread into white bread. However, you're better off with the whole grain. Grains provide protein, fiber, and healthful complex carbs.
- **Fruits:** Fruit can be a snack, a dessert, or, for that matter, a meal. Blueberries, papayas, mangoes, apples, oranges, bananas, pears, and zillions of other varieties are vitamin-rich and, like all plant foods, free of animal fat and essentially free of cholesterol, too.

To see how these four simple food groups translate into meals, let's have dinner at an upscale Italian restaurant. The waiter lights the candles and offers you a glass of wine, which you can accept or not. Then he brings a plate of grilled bread topped with diced tomatoes, basil, and a touch of garlic, and we then debate whether it is pronounced brushetta or brusketta. Our waiter assures us that there is indeed a "k" sound in bruschetta.

Next up, a choice of lentil soup, minestrone, or pasta e fagioli—a delightfully rich bean-and-pasta soup—followed by a spinach salad with cherry tomatoes, cucumbers, sliced almonds, herbs, and a light balsamic vinaigrette.

So, let's check our score. Lentils are a legume. Spinach is a vegetable. Bread and pasta are grains. And we haven't seen any meat or cheese on anything. So far, so good.

Just when we thought there could be no more appetizers, the chef tells us he has just received a shipment of poivrade artichokes from France. They are violet-tinged and smaller than the globe artichokes we are familiar with. He has cooked them in a light white wine and vegetable broth, and they are delicious. Another one for the vegetable category.

The chef has next sent us angel hair pasta topped with a spicy arrabbiata sauce, served with grilled asparagus and sides of broccoli with sautéed garlic.

If you have room for dessert, you have a choice of soy chocolate pudding, vanilla berry sorbet, sliced mandarin oranges, or blueberries.

The next day, we try a similar adventure at lunch, but we'll go Mexican. Start with a green salad, and then choose the bean burrito, the spinach enchilada, or the vegetable fajitas. Or we could have sampled foods from China, Japan, Thailand, India, or just about anywhere else, and have found delights drawn from four healthful food groups: vegetables, fruits, whole grains, and legumes.

What's Out

So the healthful staples are vegetables, fruits, whole grains, and legumes. What are the problem foods?

The problem foods are those that dump fat (especially saturated fat), cholesterol, sodium, animal proteins, and added oils and sugars on your plate. These foods contribute to weight gain, cholesterol and blood pressure problems, diabetes, and all manner of other health issues, from asthma to migraines.

We've already talked about the issues with cheese. It is loaded with fat, which means lots of unwanted calories. And most of the fat is *saturated* fat, which, along with cheese's load of cholesterol, boosts "bad cholesterol" in your bloodstream. Cheese is also high in sodium, which is tough on blood pressure, and its proteins can trigger inflammatory problems. In a word, cheese is trouble. But it is not the only problem food. Here are the foods to avoid:

- **Dairy products:** Some dairy products are fatty, others are high in sensitizing proteins, and many have both of these traits. It pays to avoid them all. In the fatty category are cheese, whole milk, full-fat yogurt, butter, etc. In the protein-heavy category are the skim and fat-free products. Many people find that, once they break free from dairy products, their health takes a turn for the better.

- **Eggs:** Eggs have a huge load of cholesterol (in the yolk) and animal protein (in the white). You do not need animal protein at all; you will get more than enough protein from plant-based foods. And, like dairy products, eggs have their share of "bad fat," have no fiber and no complex carbohydrate, and tend to skew the diet in an unhealthful direction.

- **Meat, poultry, and fish:** Meats are, needless to say, animal muscles. And that means they are perfect for moving a cow's legs, a chicken's wings, or a fish's tail, but they are not so good when it comes to nourishing the human body. Nutritionally, they are mixtures of animal protein and fat, along with cholesterol and occasional traces of fecal bacteria (salmonella, campylobacter, E. coli, etc.). Set them aside.

- **Added oils:** It pays to keep vegetable oils to a minimum, too. It is certainly true that olive oil is better than cheese or chicken fat as it has much less saturated ("bad") fat. But here are the numbers: Over 60 percent of the fat in Cheddar cheese is saturated fat. For chicken fat, the number is around 30 percent. For olive oil, it is 14 percent. So olive oil is clearly better. But there is no need to be adding *any* bad fat to your diet. Bad fat is bad for the heart and also associated with Alzheimer's risk. It is also a likely contributor to the insulin resistance that leads to type 2 diabetes.

Also, as you'll recall from Chapter 2, all fats and oils have 9 calories per gram—more than twice the calories of carbohydrates. So getting away from added fats is an easy way to trim away unwanted calories. And if particles of fat building up inside your muscle and liver cells have led to diabetes, getting away from fat is an important part of solving the problem.

Think about it: There is no faucet on an olive tree. To get a liter of olive oil, you have to take the oil from more than 1,000 olives. Just as sugar producers extract their product from sugar beets or sugar cane, oil producers throw away the pulp and fiber. In the same way that sugar is "processed" or "refined" food, extracted oils are not anything that nature ever dreamed up.

So keeping oils low is a good idea. This is not a zero-fat diet, however. Surprising as it may sound, there are traces of natural fats in all plant foods. If you were to send a leaf of spinach or a pound of beans to a laboratory, you would learn that, indeed, these foods contain traces of fats. They have nowhere near the fat content of meats, dairy products, or eggs, but they do have traces of fat, and that is good. They provide the good fats your body needs.

There are a few plant-based foods that are high in fat: Nuts, seeds, olives, avocados, and some soy products have substantial amounts of fat. If you are trying to lose weight or tackle diabetes, I would encourage you to keep them to a minimum.

- **Sugary, processed foods:** The natural sugars found in fruits are healthful and nutritious. They provide glucose that powers your brain, your muscles, and all the rest of you. They are foods we were designed to be eating.

  But added sugar—the sweetener in soda, the sugar in cookies, etc.—is not health food. In modest quantities, it is not worth worrying about—a teaspoon of sugar has only about 15 calories. But sweeteners can be added to foods in such quantities that the calories add up.

  Even so, it is good not to overstate sugar's downside. Food writers and the media have been eager to blame sugar for all manner of health problems, when much of that blame should rightly go to cheese, meat, and other greasy, unhealthy foods. Sugar simply does not have anywhere near the calories that fatty foods have, nor does it have any cholesterol or "bad fat."

  When evaluating processed foods, a handy tool is the Glycemic Index. It was invented by Dr. David Jenkins in 1981, and it helps you sort out which foods will cause your blood sugar to rise more quickly, and which foods are gentler on your blood sugar. White bread, for example, will cause your blood sugar to rise fairly quickly. It is a high-Glycemic-Index (or high-GI) food. Rye and pumpernickel breads are much gentler on your blood sugar. If you have diabetes, high triglycerides, or frequent cravings, you would do well to steer clear of high-GI foods. Here are the main ones, along with easy replacements:

- **Table sugar:** To state the obvious, sugar you eat causes your blood sugar to rise. Fruits are a better choice. Even though they are sweet, they are surprisingly gentle on your blood sugar.

- **White and wheat breads:** Something about wheat bread causes a steeper blood sugar rise than most other grains. Rye and pumpernickel breads have lower GI values. Surprisingly, however, wheat *pasta* (as opposed to wheat bread) does not have a high Glycemic Index. Unlike light, fluffy bread, pasta is so compacted that it digests slowly.

- **White potatoes:** Large white potatoes tend to make blood sugar rise quickly, while sweet potatoes are much gentler on your blood sugar.

- **Most cold cereals:** Typical children's cereals break apart quickly in the digestive tract, releasing sugars into your bloodstream. Oatmeal and bran cereal are better choices.

Supplements

Although most of your nutrition should come from foods, there are two supplements that I recommend.

Vitamin B_{12} is essential for healthy nerves and healthy blood. It is not made by animals or plants. It is made by bacteria. The body needs only a tiny amount—about 2.4 micrograms per day. Some people speculate that, before the era of modern hygiene, the bacteria in the soil, on our vegetables, on our fingers, and in our mouths produced the traces of B_{12} we need. However, those sources are not reliable today, if they ever were. Meat-eaters get traces of B_{12} produced by bacteria in an animal's intestinal tract. But not only is that not a healthful source, the B_{12} in meat is not necessarily easy to absorb. People who produce relatively little stomach acid, people on acid-blocking medications, people on metformin for diabetes, and many other people tend to run low in B_{12}. That is why the U.S. government recommends B_{12} supplements for everyone over age fifty. I would go further and recommend it for everyone, period—regardless of age.

If you follow a plant-based (vegan) diet, as I recommend, a B_{12} supplement is not optional—it is essential. That means a daily multivitamin (choose a brand that does *not* have added iron or copper), B complex, or just plain B_{12}. You will find it in any drugstore or health food store. Adults need just 2.4 micrograms per day, and all common brands have more than this. There is no danger from higher doses.

Vitamin D normally comes from sun on your skin. About fifteen or twenty minutes of sun on your face and arms will give you a good daily dose. Vitamin D helps you absorb calcium from the foods you eat and appears to have an anti-cancer effect, too.

Unfortunately, our forebears had the bad judgment to leave tropical Africa and move to places like Reykjavik, Fargo, and New York, which means it is too darn cold to go outside some of the time. So if you are mostly indoors—or if you use a sunscreen, which is good advice, too—you'll want to take a vitamin D supplement. A daily supplement of about 2,000 IU per day is safe and helpful. Higher doses can be dangerous and should be used only when directed by a physician.

There are many other supplements, but I generally do not recommend them. Some people take DHA—the ingredient of interest in fish oil. It is available now in vegan versions, which are free of the concerns about fish sources. Doses of 100 to 300 milligrams per day are likely safe. However, some people note a tendency toward bleeding when they take higher doses of DHA (something that can also occur with high fish intake), so be cautious.

I would recommend *against* taking beta-carotene or vitamin E supplements. The reason is that beta-carotene is one member of a group of cancer-fighting compounds called *carotenoids.* If you take beta-carotene alone, your body may have a harder time absorbing the other natural carotenoids. Similarly, foods naturally contain eight different forms of vitamin E. If you take a supplement that has just one or two, they can interfere with your absorption of the others. Beta-carotene and vitamin E are both available naturally in foods along with the other nutrients your body needs, so supplementing is unnecessary.

I would also recommend against taking calcium tablets, unless your physician has specifically recommended them for you. The reason is that an overly high calcium intake is associated with prostate cancer in men, as we saw in Chapter 4. Whether there is an analogous risk in women is not yet clear. Calcium-rich green leafy vegetables and beans are fine, but the concentrated calcium in pills—or, for that matter, in dairy products—has been linked to cancer.

How Healthful Foods Work

Here is how these simple foods work their magic on specific health concerns:

- **Weight loss:** A plant-based diet is powerful for weight control. First of all, beans, vegetables, fruits, and whole

grains have lots of fiber, and fiber has effectively no calories, but is filling. That means it tricks the brain into thinking you've eaten a lot, when you have actually eaten a
more reasonable portion of food. In addition, plant-based
foods increase your after-meal metabolism, giving you an
extra "burn" for a few hours after every meal.

- **Lowering cholesterol:** There is very little saturated
  fat and effectively no cholesterol in a plant-based diet.
  So your cholesterol level is likely to fall substantially. In
  addition, certain foods have an extra cholesterol-lowering
  effect. This has been demonstrated with oats, beans, soy
  products, and several other plant-based foods.

- **Reducing blood pressure:** A plant-based diet is high
  in potassium, which lowers blood pressure, and also
  reduces the thickness (viscosity) of the blood. These factors, along with the gradual weight loss the diet change
  can bring, will often cause blood pressure to fall significantly and greatly reduce the need for medication.

- **Diabetes:** As I mentioned above, a low-fat plant-based
  diet improves insulin sensitivity, presumably because
  it helps the body eliminate the fat particles that hinder
  insulin action. The improvement in blood sugar control
  can be dramatic, reducing the need for medications and
  sometimes making the disease disappear altogether.

- **Arthritis, migraines, respiratory problems, and skin
  conditions:** For many conditions, the elimination of sensitizing proteins, especially dairy proteins, leads to the
  dramatic improvements you have read about in this book.

This list is just a brief summary of the potential benefits of a
healthful diet. You'll find much more information about putting

foods to work in my previous books and at the Physicians Committee's website, PCRM.org.

Putting It All Together

Natasha grew up in Melbourne, Australia, with a mother, a father, a brother, and lots and lots of allergies. Her father had hay fever, as did her brother. For her mother, the problem was eczema, an inflammatory skin condition that was so itchy she scraped her legs with a wire sponge—the kind used for dishes—to the point where she started to bleed.

Natasha inherited all of it. Chronically congested, she had a runny nose more or less all day and all night. Her mother would come into her bedroom in the morning to find the floor covered with tissues. Skin testing showed allergies to pollen, dust, cat and dog dander, and practically everything else, and that was exactly what she experienced. If she cuddled too much with Lily, her Maltese Shih Tzu, she started sneezing. And eventually her allergies turned into asthma.

Being stuffed up and congested is not helpful for anyone. But it was especially a problem for Natasha. She was a radio journalist and had to sound clear, bright, and energetic. She took antihistamines and inhaled steam, but these did not cure her. A doctor recommended surgery to widen her nasal passages, but the prospects of success were limited and the potential risks were daunting.

Just as she had her father's allergies, she had her mother's eczema—red, itchy, dry patches behind her knees, inside her elbows, and on her hands and cheeks—and it flared up when she was stressed. A cortisone-based cream helped some, but it was clearly no cure.

One day, she and her husband Luca decided to make a

change in their lives. Working in radio, then in corporate communications, she felt there had to be something more meaningful than advertising commercial products. Luca felt the same way. He had a career in banking, but wanted to measure life in something other than currency. So they began a series of travels to explore the world, which led them not only to different cultures but also to different foods. A three-month stay in India led to a vegetarian diet, and eventually they decided to set aside dairy products and eggs, too. And suddenly, things started to improve. Her eczema disappeared. Even when she was stressed, her skin was fine. Menstrual pains that had bothered her for years disappeared, too. And although she had never been overweight, she found that the new way of eating kept her a touch leaner than before—all good changes.

But her allergies were still a problem. Time for one more tune-up. As she had gotten away from cheese and other fatty animal products, she had replaced them with equally fatty plant products, adding avocados, coconut oil, and olive oil to her salads, and eating large amounts of various nut- and seed-based foods. In theory, these were "healthy fats," but she was having a lot of them. How about ditching those extra-fatty foods?

They gave it a try. Instead of fatty snacks and oily foods, they enjoyed bananas and other fresh fruit, and started preparing meals *sans* grease. They enjoyed this new, lighter menu and the energy it gave them.

Then one evening at dinner, Luca asked, "Have you noticed something?" They looked at each other, and it hit her. She was breathing perfectly normally—and had been for a couple of days. No allergies, no sneezing, no wheezing, no coughing, no asthma. This was remarkable. They stuck with it, and she continued to feel really well.

A month later, they took a trip to Peru to see the sights,

including Machu Picchu, the ancient city of the Incas. At 7,970 feet above sea level, it is a place where tourists need to take it slow and easy. But Natasha and Luca felt good and strong. They ran uphill, fueled by exuberance and open, clear lungs. Reaching the top, Natasha cried. The chains that had kept her from living a normal life had finally been broken.

From now on, it was out with the grilled cheese and ice cream, but also out with fatty replacements. They fell in love with simple foods: a breakfast of oatmeal with cinnamon and bananas, a lunch of roasted potatoes with beans, or lentil and rice dishes, with plenty of fresh fruit.

And they took one last step, which was to let others know about the answers they had found. They made videos about their experiences and launched a YouTube channel, called "That Vegan Couple." And they began to hear from people all over the world who were as surprised as they were to learn of the power of simple diet changes.

Two Steps for Getting Started

Ready for a diet change? It's actually surprisingly easy. We have developed a two-step approach in our research studies with hundreds of people, and I have never heard of anyone unable to do this:

Step 1: Check out the possibilities. Don't change your diet yet. You're not ready. Instead, take a week or so to see what foods you might like. I suggest you take a piece of paper and write down four categories: breakfast, lunch, dinner, and snacks. Then, over the next week, jot down foods that are free of animal products and fit into each category. The idea is to find foods you like. You'll find many ideas in the recipe section (page 197).

Step 2: Do a three-week test drive. Once you've found the foods you like, put a healthy diet to a three-week test. For twenty-one days, have your diet be 100 percent plant-based, choosing from the foods you already know you like. Don't set a foot wrong. Really do it, so you can see how you feel. If you like how you're feeling, stick with it.

Jump In!

There is nothing quite like the feeling of being healthy and in control. Now that you know how a healthful diet works, let me encourage you to give it a try. The next chapter will give you lots of great ways to start.

CHAPTER 10

All the Flavor, None of the Regrets

Arriving in Rome for a scientific conference, I was not sure that any restaurants would still be open. It was late. But the Eternal City lived up to its name, and the streets were bustling with tourists and late-night diners. Smeraldo was a small, friendly restaurant, and its menu had something you would never see in Minneapolis: a pizza with no cheese at all. It was topped with fresh herbs, veggies, and a splash of olive oil, but not a speck of cheese. It was the same at the other pizzerias. Although most pizzas had cheese, every restaurant seemed to have at least one or two made without it. And when cheese was used, it was never slathered on like asphalt, the way it is in the United States.

The lesson here is that cheese is not the sine qua non of great culinary traditions—not in Rome or anywhere else. You will dine perfectly well—in fact, better—without it. In this chapter, I will show you how.

We will look at how to replace cheese in pizzas, lasagna, and other Italian-style dishes, as well as in sandwiches, toppings for salads and vegetables, snacks with crackers or bread, and desserts. Although cheese may call your name for a little while as you're leaving it behind, you will soon come to prefer the foods that replace it. They are lighter, more delicate, and much more healthful.

Let's start with a look at a number of delightful nondairy cheeses that have arrived on store shelves. Then we will look at pizza toppings, sandwich fillings, and everything else.

Plant-Based Cheese

The Right Combination

Michael Schwarz, whom we met in Chapter 7, jumped in the culinary deep end. He set out to make a delicious cheese without a drop of milk. Others had found handy ways to get a cheese taste using nutritional yeast and other ingredients, as we will see below and in the recipe section of this book. But Michael wanted to go a step further—to use the actual cheese-making process—bacterial cultures, fermentation, and all—to produce a cheese with no animal ingredients.

Michael was not a chef. He was a lawyer who was much more comfortable with patents, trademarks, copyrights, and trade secrets than bacterial cultures and fermentation vats. But he knew how to approach a problem, and he aimed to succeed.

Cheese makers have used kinds of milk from cows, goats, sheep, and water buffalos, along with all manner of bacterial strains to try to get the right texture and taste. But now the process had to work with a product that wasn't milk at all. "It's not easy to do," Michael said. "I started experimenting with various nuts and a variety of cultures. The first experiments didn't work at all. But eventually I stumbled on the answer."

The winning formula was to make a cream from cashews and inoculate it with just the right amount of *Lactobacillus acidophilus* to produce the fermentation that creates the taste of cheese. A soft cheese, perfect for spreading on crackers, could be made with a short fermentation. By adding herbs, garlic, or chipotle and serrano peppers, Michael gave each of his cheeses a unique personality. For harder varieties, Michael aged his cheeses to produce a sliceable finished product that could hold its own on any cheese plate.

The cheese that had debuted in a small Long Island town became a hit. Store after store began offering Treeline cheeses throughout the U.S. And soon it will be sold in Europe, hopefully including Germany, where Michael's story began. In the country his father had fled, he is looking forward to selling a cheese specifically designed to be free of cruelty.

Miyoko's Magic

A short drive north of the Golden Gate Bridge, Miyoko Schinner works magic. Miyoko was born in a small Japanese village between Tokyo and Yokohama. There were not many cars in her village, and there was no cheese at all. Rice and vegetables were their staple foods, not grilled cheese sandwiches. The daughter of an American father and a Japanese mother, she moved with her family to the San Francisco Bay Area at age seven. And there, she discovered some new things.

Like pizza. At a friend's house, she had her first taste. And it was...

"*Disgusting!*" Miyoko said. "Japanese foods are very light. But this had grease dripping all over it, and I almost choked."

As time went by, however, her taste buds were slowly but surely seduced. Americans liked the greasy, heavy taste of pizza, and she began to like it, too.

When she was twelve, her tastes took another turn. She went on a camping trip with a group of children who were vegetarian. They talked about animals and ethical issues, as well as youngsters can. When she got home, a slice of pork had completely lost its appeal. She couldn't eat it. "I began to feel that I would no more eat a piece of a pig or cow than I would eat a piece of a desk. It was just not food anymore." And there and then, she stopped eating meat.

This idea did not go over so well with her parents. Her mother let her know that, if she was going to eat that way, she'd have to cook for herself. And so that is what she did. Miyoko started to learn her way around the kitchen.

"The first recipe I tried was just stewed tomatoes, kidney beans, and onions. But it actually turned out very well. And I started cooking more and more, and eventually my mother started asking me to cook for the family."

In high school, Miyoko plowed through the Time-Life *Good Cook* series from start to finish, finding ways to replace the animal products she had crossed off her shopping list.

Although she avoided meat, she continued eating cheese and other dairy products for a while. But she had frequent stomach pains and digestive problems. So she decided to see how life was without these indulgences. She threw out the dairy products, and her stomach issues quickly resolved.

After college, she returned to Japan and continued to refine her culinary skills. The country has a surprising number of Michelin-starred restaurants, and she jumped into high-end cuisine, digging into every French and Italian cookbook she could get her hands on, adapting them to her now meatless and dairy-less palate.

"I went through *Mastering the Art of French Cooking* and tried to make vegan versions of everything," she said. "I wanted to prove to the world that you could still have these wonderful foods."

She applied traditional culinary techniques to entirely plant-based ingredients, inviting people to try her creations at twelve-course dinner parties. They were impressed. "Next thing I knew I was in magazines and teaching, and demonstrating products for companies." She opened a wholesale bakery and delivered her wares all over Tokyo. Then, in 1989 she returned to San Francisco, opened a bakery and a restaurant, and began writing cookbooks, including *Artisan Vegan Cheese.*

Today, her company, Miyoko's Kitchen, offers a surprising array of vegan cheese delights. Her Aged English Smoked Farm-house has the flavor of wild hickory—wild, as in uncultivated, grown by nature with no pesticides or anything else. "People say it's just like a smoked Gouda. But I wasn't trying to replicate Gouda. We're not making Cheddar or Gruyère. We are creating new styles that stand on their own."

Miyoko also sells Mt. Vesuvius Black Ash, whose color comes from a coating of ash from maritime pine, grown in southern France. The black ash coating raises the pH on the surface of the wheel, helps dry it out, and creates a smooth texture. Over time, the bacteria in the cheese release carbon dioxide bubbles, making tiny holes in the ash, and flavors become more complex.

Miyoko's Fresh Loire Valley in a Fig Leaf is a delight for the eye and the taste buds. Using a traditional French technique, she macerates fig leaves in an organic white California wine, then wraps them around the wheel to impart a special flavor of their own. But you'll only find it between May and early October, when there are fig leaves to be had.

And how do you eat it? "Just nibble on it," Miyoko says. "A little goes a long way."

Taking Nondairy Cheese to the Next Level

Tal Ronnen decided to take the world of plant-based cheeses to a new level, and he had the team to do it. Tal runs Crossroads—*the* place to be in LA, with high-end cuisine, an entirely vegan menu, and more celebrities per square inch than an Academy Awards green room. In 2011, Tal formed a new company, Kite Hill, to make nondairy cheeses.

The team included renowned Stanford biochemist Patrick Brown; Monte Casino, who had taught artisan cheese making at Le Cordon Bleu; Jean Prevot, an engineer who had overseen traditional cheese-making operations in France, Hungary, and the U.S., and was ready for a new challenge; and Matthew Sade, an innovative entrepreneur and business leader.

Cheese starts with milk, and that's where the team looked first. How do you make a milk—without a cow or goat or a buffalo—that will support the right kind of fermentation, form the right kind of curd, and ultimately give you the texture and flavor you want?

The answer was almonds. In the same way that almond milk splashes on cereal as well or better than cow's milk, it can be turned into cheese, too—at least in theory. Except that the balance of protein and fat that works in a glass of milk is not necessarily the blend that will make bacteria happy in the fermentation process or that works optimally as cheese ages. So the team tested twenty-six different almond varieties before hitting on the right one, and then let the traditional cheese-making process take it from there.

After months of experimenting, Tal, Patrick, and Monte got together in Boston with a wheel of their new product and some fresh sourdough bread. And the three of them were blown away.

The team perfected its soft fresh original, then made a variety with truffle oil, dill, and chives, and a soft ripened cheese. They then made a ricotta to go into ravioli along with either mushrooms or spinach, plus a cheesecake, a pumpkin cheesecake tart, cream cheese, and yogurt.

Tal is constantly innovating. But although he always has his sleeves rolled up, there's never a worried look on his brow. "When you love something, it doesn't feel like a job," he said.

For a diehard dairy cheese eater, plant-based cheeses are not quite the same as animal-derived varieties, just as cheese from a goat is not the same as cheese from a cow, and raw-milk cheeses are not the same as pasteurized products. But for aroma, taste, mouthfeel, and everything else that matters, plant-based cheeses have proven that cows and goats are no more necessary for cheese making than horses are for pulling wagons.

Putting It All Together at Sublime

We have been looking at how creative culinary minds approach their craft. All these innovations come together at Sublime, the legendary Fort Lauderdale night spot. As you walk in the door, you realize this is no ordinary restaurant and bar. Nanci Alexander built it from the ground up—waterfalls, original Peter Max paintings, and all—and it has attracted a long list of celebrity patrons.

At the bar, chicly dressed diners are sipping tiramisu martinis, Irish coffee, mojitos, Sublime Sunsets, and Moscow Mules. Opening the menu, you discover a stunningly creative range of flavors. Start with freshly baked Florentine Flatbread. Topped with sautéed baby spinach and onions, shredded vegan mozzarella, and tomato, and popped in the oven, it could be a meal by itself. Make a mental note to try the Roasted Vegetable Flatbread on your next trip to Sublime to see how the red peppers, squash, zucchini, olives, basil, sun-dried tomatoes, vinaigrette, plus vegan mozzarella and tomato match up.

Then, how about an appetizer or two? Mac 'n' Cheese is delicious and familiar, served in a cute bowl. The melted Cheddar is entirely plant-based. Ditto for the Cheddar on the sliders—those mini burgers on mini buns. And share a spinach salad or Caesar salad, if you like.

For a main dish, try the Mushroom Ravioli. The cheese—made from raw cashews—is blended with mushrooms, and the result is light and delicate. If you have a bigger appetite, you might go for the lasagna. Instead of cow's milk cheese, it's made with soy mozzarella, tofu, and nutritional yeast and is hearty and flavorful.

Whatever you do, save room for the cheesecake—strawberry, pumpkin, or Key lime, depending on the season. And, yes, that's a soy-based cream cheese. Want it à la mode? The vanilla ice cream is made in house, of course, and is dairy-free.

Every single item is made without a shred of cheese or any other animal product. And yet this restaurant seduces the most ardent carnivore. "Most of our clients are meat-eaters," Nanci said. "They came with a friend or heard about our food, and night after night, they thank me for what we've built."

Doing It at Home

Feeling inspired? You might not be ready to produce a fine aged cheese coated with black ash from a maritime pine or wrapped in a fig leaf. But you can create killer pasta dishes, serve up pizza that is the center of the party, make inspired sandwiches, and finish salads with flavorful toppings—all with healthful, entirely nondairy ingredients. Let's see how, with the help of Dreena Burton, the master cook who developed the recipes for this book.

Pizza Toppings

Let's start with pizza. When I was in college my friends and I drove to Chicago and ate at Pizzeria Uno, a restaurant that was unassuming except for the fact that its pizza was unlike any other, served in a deep dish and slathered with what seemed like an inch of mozzarella. We had never seen such a thing. It was gooey and indulgent, and one pizza could have fed an army. Pizzeria Uno was a hit, spawning Pizzeria Due, and eventually turning into a remarkably successful franchise.

But enough was enough. Other pizza chains followed suit, piling cheese higher and higher, and what had been a culinary curiosity became routine. Along the way, whatever delicacy pizza might have had was forgotten.

It's time to degrease the pizza. Here are some simple, tasty steps to build your own pizza *senza formaggio*:

1. Start by letting the herbs and spices speak for themselves. As we saw in the Rome pizzerias, pizza with herbs and no cheese at all is an Italian tradition, and it can be yours, too. Traditional favorites are basil, oregano, rosemary, smoked paprika—either in the crust or sprinkled into the sauce—and you can keep it as light as you like.
2. Next, think about your sauce. There are plenty of commercial brands available. But you can make your own with simple tomato paste, some dried basil and oregano, a splash of balsamic vinegar, and a touch of maple syrup, sea salt, and black pepper. See page 248 for the recipe.

3. Do your veggies right. Some restaurants throw raw onions, green peppers, cheese, and sauce on a cheap crust, singe it in the oven, and plunk down a pizza that is half-baked in every sense of the term. Don't do that. Here are better ways to do your vegetable toppings. First, be choosy about what goes on top:

- Sautéed or roasted onions: Cooking onions before they go into the oven softens their bite and adds a touch of natural sweetness. In Saint-Tropez in the French Riviera—the village made famous by Brigitte Bardot and filmmakers of the 1950s—everyone stops at Pizzeria Bruno for an informal meal with friends. Delicately sautéed onions add just the right touch to their pizza.

- Garlic: Finely chopped raw garlic will work, but browning it for a few minutes in a pan will tame its wild side before you add it to your pizza. Or, try roasted garlic. You can roast it at home or buy roasted garlic cloves at your grocery deli. What you don't use right away can be refrigerated or frozen for later use.

- Mushrooms: Not just button mushrooms. Try portobello, cremini, or shiitake mushrooms for more robust flavors. Lightly sauté, grill, or roast them to draw out extra moisture and concentrate flavors.

- Grilled or roasted vegetables: Think zucchini, eggplant, and bell peppers.

- Spinach: Either fresh or lightly cooked and well drained, or sautéed chopped kale.

- Cooked potatoes: It may seem odd to add potatoes to a pizza, but they are delicious and hearty. Use parboiled or leftover cooked potatoes. Slice or cube and add to pizza. And next, try sweet potatoes!

- Olives: Go for kalamata, black, green, or any other variety. Extra points if you remove the pits in advance.
- Sun-dried tomatoes.
- Capers.
- Artichoke hearts: Choose the water-packed (not oil-packed) hearts, and dice them first.
- Jalapeños: Dice and sprinkle on top.
- Pineapple chunks.

4. Then, coming out of the oven, add:
   - Fresh basil leaves.
   - Avocado slices or cubes.
   - Chopped chives or thinly sliced green onions.
   - Balsamic reduction: A drizzle of concentrated balsamic vinegar adds a delicious flavor (see page 215).
   - Avocado cream or cashew cream: If you are not using a dairy cheese substitute, a drizzle of either of these creams will add richness and coolness to offset the pungent, concentrated ingredients on pizza. See the recipes on page 212.
   - Nutritional yeast: Sprinkle it on. Nutritional yeast adds a light, cheese-like flavor to sauces with no fat and practically no calories. Try it! You'll find it in health food stores. Note that it is not the same as baker's yeast or brewer's yeast, which have a bitter flavor.

5. Or try some vegan cheeses. Yes, a sprinkling of herbs, a light sauce, well-prepared vegetables, and a bit of nutritional yeast will make a bang-up great pizza. But if you like, you will find dairy-free cheeses—including meltable varieties—at health food stores and many regular groceries, ready to go on your pizza. Be sure to read the ingredients list; a quirk of the labeling laws allows cheeses

to call themselves "nondairy" or "dairy-free" even when casein—the dairy protein—is one of the first ingredients. So, if your migraines or joint pain are triggered by dairy products, these substitutes will not help.

Italian Pastas

Lasagna and ravioli without cheese? *Magnifico!* They are lighter and tastier than the cheesy versions. Try our Spinach–Sweet Potato Lasagna (page 251). Or modify your favorite recipes, using the cheese substitutes I'll describe here. If you're hosting a party or bringing a dish to a potluck, you'll hit a home run with spinach lasagna or mushroom ravioli. Everyone loves them, including children and anyone who is thinking *flavor.*

For any pasta that features ricotta, try using our Tofu "Ricotta" (page 222), Tangy Cashew "Cheese" (page 219), Tofu "Feta" (page 217), Soy-Free "Feta" (page 218), or even the "Cream Cheese" (page 216) or Sour Cream 'n' Onion "Cream Cheese" (page 216). And why not break up a "Cheese" Ball (pages 223–225) to crumble into a pasta bake? You'll also find nondairy Parmesans and meltable cheeses at health food stores.

For manicotti, make a filling with the Tofu "Ricotta" and cooked sweet potato or roasted red peppers or other vegetables. Top your spaghetti or angel-hair pasta with our So-Simple Lentil Pasta Sauce (page 249) or "Parmesan" (page 220). And don't miss our Luscious Fettuccine Alfredo (page 242) and our Mac 'n' Trees (page 246) featuring broccoli or cauliflower florets.

If you're feeling pressed for time or just don't feel like cooking, health food stores and many regular grocery stores now stock a variety of frozen nondairy Italian dishes—lasagna, ravioli, pizza, and many others.

Salad Toppings

Let's make a salad special. You don't need Parmesan or feta. Instead, try these salad enhancers that are lighter, healthier, and better overall:

- Nondairy cheese: Our Tofu "Feta" (page 217) and Soy-Free "Feta" (page 218) take advantage of the savory flavor of miso, with a little vinegar, garlic, and a few other ingredients. Wonderful on a salad! Or, if you want to keep it super-simple, pick up some baked tofu at a health food store. Just cut it up, and add to a salad. Our "Parmesan" (page 220), made with cashews or almonds, and Nut-Free "Parmesan" (page 221) offer extra flavor to salads.

- Avocado chunks: Avocados have the mouthfeel, flavor, and substance that can make a salad come alive. At the store, choose avocados with a dark-green color and a little give when you press them. If the store does not have ripe avocados, just pick up a few and keep on the countertop for a few days. Once ripe, refrigerate the extra avocados to extend their freshness. One note of caution: Avocados have a healthier *kind* of fat than you'll find in cheese; like olives, they have mostly *monounsaturated* fat, rather than the *saturated* fat that predominates in cheese. But they are not a low-fat food. So if you're aiming to lose weight or tackle diabetes, avocados join the other fatty foods in the let's-avoid-them-for-now department.

- Olives: Sliced or whole in any variety, olives add flavor and color. Try kalamata, green, or dry Moroccan olives.

- Exotic fruit: Sliced papaya, mangoes, pineapples, grapes, kiwi, lychees, tangerines, cherries—you name it. They all

add a special look and flavor. And go seasonal, with blueberries, raspberries, and strawberries in summer, grapes
in the fall, and persimmons, clementines, or pomegran-
ate seeds in the winter.

- Dried fruit: Drop in raisins, dried cranberries, chopped
dried apricots, goji berries, dried blueberries, and more.
Just a small amount will add a sweet and chewy contrast
to the other salad ingredients.

- Canned vegetables: Artichoke hearts, bamboo shoots,
or sliced lotus root make a salad special and visually
appealing.

- Savory nuts and seeds: A sprinkling of chopped pecans
or walnuts, sliced almonds, pine nuts, cashews, chopped
Brazil nuts, pistachios, pumpkin seeds, sesame seeds, or
sunflower seeds add flavor, not to mention vitamin E.
Toast them just slightly, and you'll get more flavor with
smaller servings.

- Chickpeas: Try our roasted Greek Chickpeas (page 226)
or black beans to boost the protein content and make a
salad more like a meal.

- Plant-based "bacon": Foods like eggplant, mushrooms,
seaweed, and coconut have all found their place in
plant-based "bacon" products! Coconut bacon is most
popular now, and it's easy to find store-bought varieties.
Or make your own with our recipe on page 232.

- Fresh herbs: Dill, cilantro, basil, parsley, and other leafy
herbs add nuance to salads.

- Pickled foods: Capers, sauerkraut, dill or sweet pickles,
or kimchi all add flavors of their own.

- Dressings: Our recipe section, starting on page 197,
includes a selection of creamy dressings that you'll want
to try. Or keep it extra simple with just a squirt of lemon

juice or drizzle of seasoned vinegar. For an Asian flavor, try seasoned rice vinegar, or go Mediterranean with balsamic. Apple cider vinegar works great, too. For a simple quick dressing, mix vinegar, soy sauce, and maple syrup.

- Croutons: Instead of store-bought croutons that are typically high in fat, try our own Oil-Free Croutons (page 231). Once you get the hang of making them, try your own favorite seasonings.

Toppings for Vegetables

Parents know that smothering broccoli or cauliflower in cheese sauce will make children eat them, and grocery store freezers stock packs of veggies with enough cheese to undo whatever benefit the vegetables might have held. Try these toppings instead:

- Nacho Dip: Our version (page 228) goes great with steamed or raw cauliflower and broccoli.
- Nutritional yeast: Our new friend nutritional yeast adds a delicious savory taste to green beans, zucchini, broccoli, cauliflower, and just about any other vegetable. Just sprinkle it on.
- Liquid aminos: A bit like soy sauce, this product from the Bragg company brings a savory flavor to kale, broccoli, and other vegetables and combines well with nutritional yeast.
- Savory seasonings: A splash of tamari or balsamic vinegar enlivens any vegetable.
- Herbamare seasoned salt: This blend of herbs, vegetables, and spices is a tasty replacement to standard salt, and great on roasted vegetables.
- Plant-based "Parmesan": See our recipe on page 220, and try it on veggies, vegetable soups, and more.

Sandwich Fillings

Grilled cheese, ham and cheese, cheeseburgers, cheese, and more cheese—for many people, sandwiches have become little more than cholesterol wrapped in bread. We can do better. Let's try some fresh ideas.

- Submarine sandwiches: It is easy to make a sandwich without meat and cheese. Pile it high with lettuce, tomato, cucumbers, onions, spinach, olives, banana peppers, and jalapeños and sprinkle it with red wine vinegar (don't forget to toast your bread first!). And if you're on the road, Subway, Quiznos, and every other sub shop is happy to do the same.

- Pesto panini: This is quick and easy. You can make a pesto in a food processor from fresh basil, roasted garlic, toasted pine nuts or walnuts, lemon juice, salt, pepper, and a little water. (Or try our Pistachio Pesto, page 250.) Spread pesto on hearty ciabatta bread and top with roasted red peppers or zucchini, sautéed sliced portobellos, or fresh or sun-dried tomatoes, then press in a hot pan.

Hummus

The Mediterranean favorite has become a worldwide staple. Made from chickpeas and tahini (pureed sesame seeds), it spreads on a sandwich like peanut butter, and you won't think about adding cheese to the top.

If you have never tried making your own hummus, you really should. Have a look at page 226. You can whip it up in a food processor in five minutes flat, and that allows you to do something that manufacturers never thought to do, which is to trim the fat content. By using just a touch of tahini, omitting the olive oil, and adding an extra splash of water to keep it smooth, you'll make the lightest, best hummus you ever tasted. Feel free to add red peppers, garlic, and anything else. If you like, you can make it from other beans, too, like black beans or cannellinis.

Now that you are the expert, how about inviting your friends to a hummus party? Just prepare a basic hummus, and encourage guests to bring their favorite mix-ins, such as diced tomatoes, minced garlic, kalamata olives, roasted red peppers, taco seasoning, pine nuts, or roasted beets.

- Romanesco spread: Lightly blend roasted red peppers, roasted garlic, artichoke hearts, toasted almonds, salt, and pepper with a little water in a food processor. Spread on bread for a quick sandwich or snack. Romanesco keeps well in the refrigerator.
- Pimento cheese: A nondairy spread is easy to make by blending together nutritional yeast, cashews, pimentos, and lemon juice.
- CLT: How about a cucumber-lettuce-and-tomato sandwich? Add a little mustard or nondairy mayo, and you're onto something. Or try grilled veggies.
- Make it Mexican: Tacos, quesadillas, burritos, and enchiladas are often drowning in cheese. It's time to let other flavors emerge. Experiment with cumin, cayenne, coriander, turmeric, paprika, onions, cilantro, and a wide variety of peppers. Add avocado, if you like. You can make a quick filling using a can of white beans, a half-cup of salsa, and a spoon of nutritional yeast. Just blend in a food processor, spread it between two flour tortillas, and heat on the stove.

Cracker Snacks

What can top a cracker without the cholesterol and fat in cheese? We've already learned about the delightful nondairy cheeses that Michael, Miyoko, and Tal invented. Here are some more possibilities:

- Hummus: We mentioned hummus as a sandwich filling. But it works great as a spread or dip, too. Stores carry endless varieties flavored with garlic, spices, basil, olives, jalapeños, pine nuts, and everything else.
- Dips: Our recipe section has many cheese replacements that you'll want to use as dips or spreads; they start on page 216: Try the Smoky Tomato–Almond "Cheese" Ball (page 224), Herbed "Cheese" Ball (page 223), "Cream Cheese" and Sour Cream 'n' Onion "Cream Cheese" (page 216), and our Tangy Cashew "Cheese" (page 219). You'll also want to try our Roasted Tomato and Garlic Chickpea Dip (page 227) and Nacho Dip (page 228).
- Olive tapenade: You'll find it in stores, but you can make your own in a processor. Blend kalamata olives with dried figs and a touch of pepper and dried thyme.
- Red peppers: Sliced roasted red peppers are simple and attractive when served with crackers.

Desserts

Can you take the cheese out of cheesecake and still have a dessert that everyone loves? You bet! Nanci did it at Sublime, and you can, too, with our delicious Divine Cheesecake (page 263 in the dessert recipes starting on page 257). While you're at it, feast your eyes on all the other desserts made without a bit of dairy: Baked Bananas (page 265), Vanilla Bean Chocolate Cake with Dreamy

Chocolate Frosting (pages 257–258), Chocolate–Peanut Butter Gelato (page 259), Caramel Banana Ice Cream (page 260), No-Bake Iced Gingerbread Bars (page 262), Chocolate Almond Macaroons (page 261), and our Dessert Cashew Cream (page 265).

Explore the possibilities! Have fun!

Dairy-Free "Cheese" Products

Dairy-free cheeses have evolved greatly over recent years. There is now a variety of plant-based cheeses to suit every need, from melting on pizza and pasta to serving on elegant cheese platters. This list includes some of the commercial cheese options that can be useful in your dairy-free kitchen. It will only continue to grow as more dairy-free cheese products emerge to suit every dietary need and palate preference.

Cheese Slices, Cheese Shreds, and Cream Cheeses

Field Roast Chao

Sliced cheeses made from a coconut base are seasoned with a fermented tofu called chao by our Vietnamese friends. With good flavors and texture, Field Roast cheese can be eaten straight from the package or melted on pizza or in grilled cheese sandwiches.

Daiya

A very popular brand with a wide range of low-allergen cheeses (made from a tapioca base rather than nuts or soy), Daiya offers cheese shreds, slices, and blocks that all melt exceptionally well. The brand has expanded its product line into cream cheeses and also convenience foods, including cheesecakes and frozen pizzas.

(continued)

Tofutti

One of the original vegan cheese brands made from a non-GMO soy base, Tofutti products are available in slices as well as a plant-based cream cheese and sour cream.

Follow Your Heart

Follow Your Heart cheese comes in shreds, blocks, and slices, as well as soy-free products, plus a dairy-free cream cheese and sour cream.

Teese

Dairy-free Teese cheeses are packaged in tubes and particularly good for sauces and dips.

Go Veggie

Go Veggie offers slices, shreds, blocks, cream cheeses, and a Parmesan substitute (see below). Note that some Go Veggie products contain casein (dairy protein) but are still labeled "lactose-free," so you will want to read the labels.

Parmesan Alternatives

Go Veggie

This Parmesan alternative is a little more processed than the nondairy Parmesan recipes here. However, it is convenient and mimics the color, taste, and texture of dairy-based grated Parmesan cheese. As noted above, some products contain casein (dairy protein) and are labeled as "lactose-free," so it pays to read labels.

Parma!

A whole-foods substitute for Parmesan uses a blend of nutritional yeast, nuts, and salt.

Artisanal Cheeses

Kite Hill

Cultured cheeses from Kite Hill are made from an almond milk base and include soft-set artisanal cheese wheels, ricotta cheese, and cream cheeses.

Miyoko's Kitchen

Miyoko's aged cashew-based cheese wheels come in a variety of flavors. You'll also find a meltable mozzarella-style cheese and a European-style cultured dairy-free butter.

Treeline

These cultured cheeses are made from a base of cashews, and come in both a spreadable texture and firmer aged cheeses.

Dr. Cow

The first aged dairy-free cheeses on the market, Dr. Cow products are made with cashews, macadamias, and Brazil nuts.

Punk Rawk Labs

A cashew-based line of aged cheeses.

Heidi Ho

These plant-based cheeses are made from cashews and hazelnuts and include spreadable cheeses, cheese blocks, nacho cheese dips, and a soy-based feta.

CHAPTER 11

Recipes

Ready to experience the best of taste *and* the best of health? These delicious recipes were prepared by Dreena Burton. Dreena is a powerhouse in the world of recipe development, and this collection will help you ramp up the nutritional power of your favorite foods, omit animal products, maximize taste, and minimize preparation time.

One quick note: Some cheese substitutes use cashews, almonds, avocados, or similar foods that have the smooth taste cheese lovers look for. The natural fats in these foods are much more healthful than dairy fat and, unlike cheese, have no cholesterol at all. That said, even healthful fats have their share of calories. So if you are aiming to lose weight or tackle diabetes, I would suggest focusing on the lower-fat recipes. For example, you can get the taste of cheese on a pizza by adding any of the vegan cheeses you'll see here, or you can also sprinkle on some fat-free nutritional yeast.

As you prepare the recipes, consider larger quantities and storing extra portions for later use. And don't forget to share. Your friends, family, and office mates would love a taste, and you can share your wisdom with them.

Bon appétit!

Ingredient Notes and Kitchen Tools

Ingredients

Here are some ingredients that may be new to you. Some are especially useful for cheese and cream replacements.

- **Coconut butter:** Made from pureed whole flesh or "meat" of the coconut, much like how nut butters are purees of nuts (example: almond butter). When coconut butter is required in a recipe, do not substitute coconut oil. Coconut butter does not need to be refrigerated. Keep it at room temperature for use in these recipes; it will be a little softer and far easier to measure.
- **Coconut milk:** Where coconut milk is specified, this means the canned variety, rather than the cartons of drinkable coconut milks now available. Regular canned coconut milk is exceptionally thick and creamy. Some of these recipes call for separation of the liquid and cream. This is easiest to do if you refrigerate the can of milk a day or two in advance. Don't shake the can before opening, just open and scoop out the thick cream. The watery liquid can then be discarded or saved for other recipe uses.
- **Miso:** Use a mild-flavored miso in our recipes. Chickpea miso is recommended. If unavailable, use a light-colored/mild miso like barley or brown rice miso.

- **Nondairy milk:** There are many choices for nondairy milks, including soy, rice, almond, oat, coconut, flax, and hemp varieties. For these recipes, the nutritional analysis has been done using plain unsweetened soy milk (unless otherwise indicated in the recipe). In general, the recipes work best with plain soy, almond, or cashew milk. Organic, non-genetically-modified varieties are widely available.

- **Nondairy yogurt:** Several varieties of dairy-free yogurts are now available, made from bases of soy, coconut, or almond. The coconut varieties tend to be sweeter and less tangy than soy. If there is a preference for a nondairy yogurt in the recipe, it is stated.

- **Silken tofu:** A smooth and silky variety of tofu sold in small, rectangular, aseptic boxes. Silken tofu becomes very smooth and creamy when blended or pureed, so it works very well in creamy recipes like desserts and smoothies. Mori-Nu silken tofu (soft and firm varieties) can be found in most grocery stores. As with soy milk, organic, non-genetically-modified varieties are commonly available.

- **Soaked nuts:** Nuts and soaked nuts are used in many of the cream and cheese recipes here. Soaking nuts like almonds and cashews makes them softer and moister, which allows them to puree more easily and produce a creamy texture. The nuts will also plump after soaking, and this will affect the measurements. So, where a recipe requires "soaked" nuts, use nuts that have already been soaked, and *then* measure.

  To soak nuts, place in a bowl of water and cover for several hours. Nuts like cashews will take three to four hours, almonds six to eight hours. The nuts will become larger after soaking, as they swell from absorbing some of the water. Drain the soaking water, and rinse the nuts. They can be stored in the fridge (after draining/rinsing) for a few days, or frozen in an airtight container for several months. It is helpful to soak more than you will need for any given recipe. They can be frozen in batches, thaw well, and then are ready for use in recipes.

- **Tiger nut butter and tiger nut flour:** Despite its name, tiger nut is not actually a tree nut. Tiger nut is actually a small root vegetable that can be processed into a butter or a flour. It is naturally gluten-free and nut-free.

Kitchen Tools

There are a few kitchen tools that are handy for many of these recipes:

- **High-speed blender:** While these are not inexpensive machines, they do pay back their investment over time. While a high-speed blender is not critical for smoothies, it really makes a difference with spreads, cheeses, and creams. You *can* make them with a standard blender, but the process is much easier, quicker, and more enjoyable with a high-speed machine. So, consider the investment if you want to make much of your dairy-free replacements at home.
- **Food processor:** If you don't have a high-speed blender, some of the recipes can be made in a food processor instead. A food processor is not as efficient for some pureeing purposes, but often it will stand in just fine. If you are shopping for a food processor, look for one with at least a 12- or 14-cup bowl.
- **Immersion blender:** This tool is useful for soups and other recipes where it's easier to puree straight in the

cooking vessel rather than transferring to a blender (and then back to the vessel). Immersion blenders are not very expensive and are very useful to have on hand.

- **Parchment paper and parchment baking cups:** Parchment is extremely helpful in baking without using oils. It allows baked goods to easily slide off the paper (or muffins/cupcakes to slip out of the cups). The paper is also great for home fries, roasting vegetables, and other cooking needs. And as a bonus: It makes cleaning up a breeze!

Breakfast and Morning Snacks

Oatmeal with Cinnamon-Sugar Apples
Serves 2

1 cup rolled oats

1½ cups water

½ cup plain or vanilla nondairy milk, plus more if needed
    and for serving

Sea salt

1 to 1½ cups diced apple (1 medium or large)

1½ tablespoons sugar

½ teaspoon ground cinnamon

Additional sweetener (coconut sugar or pure maple syrup) (optional)

Bring the oats, water, milk, and an optional pinch of salt to a boil in a
pot over high heat. Reduce the heat to low and simmer gently for 9
to 10 minutes (or longer), until the oats are fully cooked through and
softened. Remove from heat and let stand for a few minutes; the oats
will thicken more as they sit (add extra milk if needed to thin).

Meanwhile, combine the apple, sugar, cinnamon, and a pinch of
salt in a bowl and mix.

When the oats are ready, spoon the apple mixture into 2 bowls.
Top with the oatmeal, and just very slightly stir into the oatmeal,
without overmixing. Serve, topping with sweetener and milk, if
desired.

Add-Ins: Also consider adding 1 tablespoon of ground chia seeds to
the oatmeal, or finish with a sprinkle of hemp seeds.

Per serving (½ of recipe): 241 calories, 7 g protein, 46 g
carbohydrate, 17 g sugar, 4 g total fat, 13% calories from fat, 6 g
fiber, 179 mg sodium

Cinnamon-Date Granola

Makes 5 cups

4 cups rolled oats
2 teaspoons ground cinnamon
¼ teaspoon ground nutmeg
¼ teaspoon (scant) sea salt
¼ cup nut butter (such as almond butter or cashew butter)
½ cup brown rice syrup
1 teaspoon pure vanilla extract
½ cup raisins or chopped pitted dates

Preheat the oven to 300°F and line a large rimmed baking sheet with parchment paper.

In a bowl, combine the oats, cinnamon, nutmeg, and salt and mix until well combined. In another bowl, combine the nut butter with the brown rice syrup and vanilla. Add this mixture to the oats and stir to combine well. Transfer to the lined baking sheet and spread out to evenly distribute.

Bake for 27 to 28 minutes, stirring a couple of times throughout baking to ensure the mixture browns evenly. Stir in the raisins or dates and bake for another 3 to 5 minutes, until mostly crispy. (Granola will continue to crisp after cooling, so don't overbake.) Let cool completely. Once cool, store in an airtight container. Keeps for one to two weeks.

Variation: For a festive twist, add 2 tablespoons pumpkin seeds to the oat mixture, substitute ⅓ cup dried cranberries for the dates, and add 1 teaspoon grated orange zest with the cranberries during the last minutes of baking.

Per 1-cup serving: 489 calories, 12 g protein, 87 g carbohydrate, 30 g sugar, 11 g total fat, 20% calories from fat, 9 g fiber, 145 mg sodium

Lemon-Berry Pancakes

Makes 12 pancakes (4 servings)

Serve as is with pure maple syrup, or with Dessert Cashew Cream (page 265) or Raspberry Dessert Sauce (page 264).

2 cups plus 2 tablespoons oat flour

⅓ cup rolled oats

1 tablespoon ground chia seeds

1 tablespoon baking powder

Pinch sea salt

½ teaspoon grated lemon zest

1½ teaspoons freshly squeezed lemon juice

2 cups vanilla nondairy milk (plus more if needed, see Note)

1 cup frozen or fresh raspberries, blackberries, or blueberries

In a large bowl, combine the flour, rolled oats, and ground chia. Sift in the baking powder, then add the salt. Stir to combine. Add the lemon zest, juice, and milk and whisk until combined. Add the berries and gently stir to incorporate.

Lightly oil a nonstick skillet (simply wipe oil onto the pan using a paper towel; if you have a very good nonstick pan you won't need much). Heat the pan over medium-high heat for a few minutes, until hot. Reduce the heat to medium or medium-low and let rest for a minute. Using a ladle, scoop ¼- to ⅓-cup portions of the batter into the skillet. Cook the pancakes for several minutes, until small bubbles form on the outer edges and in the centers, and the pancakes start to look dry on the top. (Wait until those bubbles form, or the pancakes will be tricky to flip.) Once ready, flip the pancakes and lightly cook on the other side, about a minute. Repeat until all the batter is used.

Milk Note: As you use up the batter, you'll notice that it becomes much thicker. So, add an extra tablespoon of milk as needed to thin the mixture as you work through batches.

Per serving (¼ of recipe): 360 calories, 15 g protein, 60 g carbohydrate, 4 g sugar, 8 g total fat, 19% calories from fat, 14 g fiber, 459 mg sodium

Chocolate Lovers' Banana Bread

Serves 10

2 cups whole-grain spelt flour
⅓ cup coconut sugar
1 tablespoon ground chia seeds
¼ teaspoon sea salt
⅓ cup cocoa powder
1½ teaspoons baking powder
½ teaspoon baking soda
1 cup pureed overripe bananas (from 2½ to 3 bananas)
¾ cup nondairy milk
⅓ cup pure maple syrup
2 teaspoons pure vanilla extract
2 to 3 tablespoons nondairy chocolate chips (optional)

Preheat the oven to 350°F. Wipe the inside of a glass loaf pan with a touch of oil on a paper towel (or use a silicone loaf pan). Use a piece of parchment paper to line the bottom and sides of the pan (makes for easy removal of the bread).

In a large bowl, combine the flour, sugar, ground chia, and salt. Sift in the cocoa, baking powder, and baking soda. Mix until well combined. In another bowl, combine the pureed bananas, milk, maple syrup, vanilla, and chocolate chips (if using). Add the wet mixture to the dry mixture and mix until just well combined.

Pour the batter into the prepared pan. Bake for 43 to 47 minutes, until the bread springs back to the touch. Transfer the pan to a cooling rack and let the bread cool completely in the pan. Lift the bread out (using the ends of the parchment) and slice.

Per serving (¹⁄₁₀ of loaf): 174 calories, 5 g protein, 38 g carbohydrate, 18 g sugar, 2 g total fat, 8% calories from fat, 5 g fiber, 205 mg sodium

Breakfast Muffins
Makes 12 large muffins

2 cups oat flour
½ cup almond meal (or tiger nut flour for a nut-free option)
1 tablespoon ground chia seeds
1½ teaspoons ground cinnamon
¼ teaspoon freshly grated nutmeg
¼ teaspoon sea salt
2 teaspoons baking powder
1 teaspoon baking soda
1 cup unsweetened organic applesauce
½ cup pure maple syrup
¼ cup plain or vanilla nondairy milk
1 teaspoon pure vanilla extract
¼ cup raisins
¼ cup dried cranberries (or other dried fruit, see Note)
1 teaspoon lemon zest (optional)
2 tablespoons rolled oats
1½ tablespoons coconut sugar

Preheat the oven to 350°F. Line 12 cups of a standard muffin pan with parchment cupcake liners.

In a large bowl, combine the oat flour, almond meal, chia, cinnamon, nutmeg, and salt. Sift in the baking powder and baking soda and mix until well combined. In another bowl, combine the applesauce, maple syrup, milk, and vanilla, and mix together. Add the wet mixture to the dry mixture. Gently fold in the dried fruit and lemon zest until just combined (do not overmix).

Spoon the batter into the muffin pan cups. Combine the rolled oats and sugar and sprinkle over the tops. Bake for 20 to 24 minutes, until a toothpick inserted in the center of a muffin comes out clean.

Dried Fruit Note: You can use all raisins (for a total of ½ cup) if you like, or try a mix of other dried fruit. Some ideas: minced dried apple, chopped apricots, chopped dates, dried blueberries, and goji berries.

Per muffin: 179 calories, 4 g protein, 33 g carbohydrate, 15 g sugar, 4 g total fat, 19% calories from fat, 4 g fiber, 241 mg sodium

Orange Apricot Tea Buns

Makes 6 buns

1½ cups oat flour

1 cup rolled oats

½ teaspoon freshly ground nutmeg

¼ teaspoon (touch scant) sea salt

1½ teaspoons baking powder

½ teaspoon baking soda

1½ teaspoons grated orange zest, or 1 teaspoon grated lemon zest (see Note)

¼ cup chopped dried unsulphured apricots or chopped pitted dates

⅓ cup freshly squeezed orange juice (juice from mandarins is also lovely!)

⅓ cup pure maple syrup

2 tablespoons plain nondairy milk

1 tablespoon ground white chia seeds

½ teaspoon pure vanilla or almond extract

Preheat the oven to 350°F. Line a baking sheet with parchment paper.

In a large bowl, combine the oat flour, oats, nutmeg, and salt. Sift in the baking powder and baking soda. Mix until well combined, then stir in the zest and apricots. In a smaller bowl, mix the orange juice, maple syrup, milk, chia, and extract. Add the wet mixture to the dry and mix until just combined. Let sit for just a minute.

Using a large cookie scoop (or a spoon), scoop out 6 portions of the batter onto the baking sheet. Bake for 14 minutes, until set to the touch. Let the buns cool for a minute on the baking sheet, then transfer to a cooling rack to cool completely.

Zest Note: Use a kitchen rasp (Microplane grater) to easily zest citrus. Be sure the citrus you use is organic, otherwise omit the zest.

Per bun: 243 calories, 6 g protein, 47 g carbohydrate, 15 g sugar, 4 g total fat, 12% calories from fat, 6 g fiber, 312 mg sodium

Fruit and Flax Breakfast Bars
Makes 16 bars

1½ cups rolled oats

½ cup oat flour

¾ teaspoon freshly grated nutmeg

¼ teaspoon sea salt

1 cup pureed overripe bananas (see Note)

⅓ cup flax meal (regular or golden flax meal)

⅓ cup pure maple syrup

2 tablespoons nondairy milk

1½ teaspoons freshly squeezed lemon juice

¼ cup pumpkin seeds or chopped nuts (such as walnuts or pecans) (optional)

3 tablespoons raisins, cranberries, or chopped dates (optional)

Preheat the oven to 350°F. Prepare an 8 x 8-inch or similar baking dish by lightly oiling the inside surface and then lining with a piece of parchment paper.

In a mixing bowl, combine the oats, oat flour, nutmeg, and salt. Add the bananas, flax meal, maple syrup, milk, and lemon juice. Mix to combine well. If you'd like to add some nuts or seeds for texture, and dried fruit for chewiness, stir those in as well.

Transfer the batter to the prepared pan and smooth with a spatula to evenly distribute. Bake for 20 minutes, until soft, moist, and set to touch but still a little soft. If you'd like them drier, bake for another 15 minutes or so, until firmer. Let cool completely in the pan. Once cool, cut into squares or bars.

Banana Note: Use a blender, or an immersion blender in a deep cup, to puree a couple of overripe bananas. If you are shy of 1 cup, make up the difference with applesauce. Or, instead of bananas, substitute a full cup of applesauce, but use 1 teaspoon ground cinnamon instead of the ¾ teaspoon nutmeg.

Per bar: 86 calories, 2 g protein, 16 g carbohydrate, 6 g sugar, 2 g total fat, 18% calories from fat, 2 g fiber, 40 mg sodium

Potato Tofu Scramble

Serves 3

1 (12- to 16-ounce) package extra-firm tofu (see Note)
1 teaspoon onion powder
½ teaspoon garlic powder
½ teaspoon black salt (kala namak, see Note)
⅛ to ¼ teaspoon sea salt (to taste, see Tofu Note)
3 tablespoons water
2½ tablespoons nutritional yeast
1 tablespoon tahini
1 tablespoon tomato paste
1½ tablespoons apple cider vinegar
1 teaspoon pure maple syrup
2 cups cubed cooked yellow or red potatoes (see Note)
3 cups (roughly) julienned kale (about 1 small bunch, stems
    removed)
⅓ cup frozen corn kernels

Use your fingers to crumble the tofu into a large nonstick skillet,
breaking it up well. Add the onion powder, garlic powder, black salt,
and sea salt and cook in the dry skillet over medium heat, stirring
occasionally, for 5 to 7 minutes.

Meanwhile, in a bowl, combine the water, nutritional yeast, tahini,
tomato paste, vinegar, and maple syrup and mix until fully combined.

Stir the yeast mixture into the tofu, then add the potatoes, kale,
and corn and mix. Continue to cook over medium heat for 5 to
7 minutes or longer, until the vegetables are heated through and
the kale has wilted. If the mixture begins to stick to the bottom, add
another splash of water and use a wooden spoon to remove any
sauce sticking to the pan. If the mixture is really sticking/scorching,
reduce the heat slightly. Taste, season as desired, and serve.

Tofu Note: If using a 16-ounce package of tofu, you may want
additional salt.

Black Salt Note: Not actually black in color, rather a light pink, black salt is sometimes labeled *kala namak*; it contributes an "eggy" flavor to dishes. If you don't have it, simply omit and season with additional sea salt to taste (using a total of ½ to ¾ teaspoon salt).

Potato Note: If you don't have any cooked potatoes, substitute 2 cups of other veggies, such as a mix of cubed frozen squash or sweet potatoes, chopped raw bell peppers, and/or halved grape tomatoes.

Add-Ins: Try adding a cup of black beans or frozen green peas with the other vegetables and cook until cooked through. For extra color, add about a half-cup of chopped bell pepper or halved grape tomatoes.

> *Per serving (⅓ of recipe):* 301 calories, 20 g protein,
> 39 g carbohydrate, 5 g sugar, 10 g total fat, 29% calories from fat,
> 7 g fiber, 575 mg sodium

Pineapple-Citrus Green Smoothie
Makes 2 large smoothies

2 cups (loosely packed) baby spinach (see Note)
1½ cups frozen pineapple cubes or chunks
½ cup thickly sliced cucumber
1 large lemon or small orange, peeled
1 to 1½ cups sliced overripe banana (frozen or fresh)
1¼ to 1½ cups water, or more to thin as desired

Optional Add-Ins
Couple tablespoons of a vanilla plant-based protein powder
2 to 3 teaspoons pure maple syrup or a pinch of stevia, to
    sweeten (optional, see Banana Note)
1 to 2 tablespoons hemp seeds

Combine the spinach, pineapple, cucumber, lemon, 1 cup banana, and 1¼ cups water in a blender, along with any optional add-ins. Puree until very smooth, adding more water as needed to puree. Taste, and if you'd like it sweeter, add the extra banana.

Spinach Note: Kale or collard greens can easily be substituted for the spinach, though they have a much stronger flavor than spinach. If you are new to green smoothies, start with just a cup of kale or collards, and then adjust to taste as you go.

Banana Note: Definitely opt for overripe (freckled) bananas. Not only are they more digestible; they also offer a great deal of natural sweetness. If the bananas aren't particularly overripe, you may want to add a touch of maple syrup to sweeten (as per the optional add-ins).

Per serving (½ of recipe): 152 calories, 3 g protein, 39 g carbohydrate, 23 g sugar, 1 g total fat, 4% calories from fat, 6 g fiber, 33 mg sodium

Blueberry Bliss Smoothie

Makes 2 large smoothies

1½ cups plain or vanilla nondairy milk, or more to thin if desired
1½ cups frozen blueberries (see Note)
1 cup sliced overripe banana (frozen or fresh)
1 cup baby spinach leaves (optional)
1 to 2 tablespoons hemp seeds
1 tablespoon pure maple syrup (optional, to sweeten if desired)

Combine all the ingredients except the maple syrup in a blender and puree for a few minutes to ensure the hemp seeds are fully pureed. Taste and add maple syrup if desired to sweeten, and extra milk to thin out if you want a thinner texture.

Berry Note: While you can use other berries here, keep in mind that the green of the spinach will only be camouflaged with the blueberries. If using red berries like strawberries or raspberries, the color will turn a brownish hue.

Per serving (½ of recipe): 237 calories, 8 g protein, 43 g carbohydrate, 25 g sugar, 6 g total fat, 22% calories from fat, 10 g fiber, 67 mg sodium

Dressings and Sauces

Luscious Cashew Cream

Makes just over 1 cup

This cream is wonderful to top potatoes, soups, casseroles, or to add to sauces and soups by the tablespoon for a touch of creaminess.

1 cup soaked raw cashews
¼ teaspoon sea salt
½ to ⅔ cup water

In a blender, puree the cashews, salt, and ½ cup water until very smooth. (A high-powered blender works best to give a very silky consistency.) For a thinner consistency, add additional water, a tablespoon at a time.

Per 2-tablespoon serving: 84 calories, 3 g protein, 5 g carbohydrate, 1 g sugar, 7 g total fat, 66% calories from fat, 0.5 g fiber, 71 mg sodium

Avocado Cream

Makes about 1¾ cups

This cream (or sauce) is spectacular with spicy dishes like chili, tacos (try Chickpea Tacos, page 245), burritos, enchiladas, and more. However, it's so luscious and creamy that you will want to try it on milder dishes as well, like cooked grains, soups, baked potatoes, pizza, and salads.

1½ cups cubed ripe avocado (1 large or 2 small avocados)
2 tablespoons freshly squeezed lemon or lime juice
½ teaspoon (scant) sea salt
½ to ⅔ cup water (to thin as desired)

Using a blender, or an immersion blender in a deep cup, puree the avocado, juice, salt, and ½ cup water until smooth. With ½ cup water, the mixture will still be fairly thick, like a cream to dollop on soup or chili. For a thinner sauce, add the additional water (or more as needed) to drizzle on pizza, burritos, salad, and more.

Leftovers Note: Avocado turns brown when exposed to the air. If you don't use all of this cream for one meal, try these tricks to minimize oxidation: (1) Transfer the cream to a deep, narrow vessel (such as a jar rather than a shallow bowl) so less of the surface area is exposed to the air. (2) Cover with plastic wrap, allowing the plastic wrap to make contact with the top of the cream (again, this reduces air exposure). (3) When serving again, simply skim off any cream that has oxidized with a spoon.

Per ¼-cup serving: 55 calories, 1 g protein, 3 g carbohydrate, 0 g sugar, 5 g total fat, 76% calories from fat, 2 g fiber, 137 mg sodium

Ranch Dressing

Makes scant 1 cup

½ cup soaked raw cashews
1 tablespoon sliced chives or green onion (green portion)
2 tablespoons apple cider vinegar
½ teaspoon Dijon mustard
¼ teaspoon garlic powder
½ teaspoon sea salt
Freshly ground black pepper, to taste
⅓ to ½ cup water
2 to 4 teaspoons pure maple syrup, to taste

In a blender, or with an immersion blender in a deep cup, blend the cashews, chives, vinegar, mustard, garlic powder, salt, pepper, ⅓ cup water, and 2 teaspoons maple syrup. If using a high-powered blender, this will smooth out very quickly. If using a standard blender/immersion blender, it will take a few minutes of blending. Once smooth, add additional water as desired to thin. Then taste, and season with additional maple syrup, salt, and/or pepper if desired. (I've found that children will enjoy the dressing more with that extra touch of maple syrup.) The dressing will thicken after refrigerating, so just thin with a little water as needed.

Per 2-tablespoon serving: 54 calories, 2 g protein, 4 g carbohydrate, 2 g sugar, 4 g total fat, 59% calories from fat, 0.5 g fiber, 166 mg sodium

Rich Tahini Dressing

Makes ¾ cup

¼ cup chickpeas or white beans
¼ cup water
3 tablespoons red wine vinegar or apple cider vinegar
2 tablespoons tahini
2 tablespoons pure maple syrup, or more to taste
1 teaspoon Dijon mustard
½ teaspoon tamari (optional, or use more salt to taste or just omit)
1 very small clove garlic, peeled (optional)
½ scant teaspoon sea salt

In a blender, or with an immersion blender in a deep cup, combine all the ingredients and puree until very smooth. Taste test, and if you'd like a touch sweeter, add more maple syrup, just ½ to 1 teaspoon at a time. This dressing will thicken after refrigerating, so just thin with a little water as needed.

Per 2-tablespoon serving: 59 calories, 1 g protein, 7 g carbohydrate, 4 g sugar, 3 g total fat, 42% calories from fat, 1 g fiber, 239 mg sodium

Sour Cream

Makes 1 cup

¾ cup plain nondairy yogurt (see Note)
½ cup soaked raw cashews
2½ teaspoons freshly squeezed lemon juice, or more to taste
¼ teaspoon (rounded) sea salt
1½ to 3 tablespoons water (adjust as needed based on yogurt, see Yogurt Note)

In a good blender (high-speed preferred), puree all the ingredients until smooth. Taste, and adjust with extra lemon juice if desired. The sour cream thickens after sitting and refrigerating.

Yogurt Note: Brands of nondairy yogurt vary in consistency. So start with 1½ tablespoons of water to blend, and add extra as desired to thin as needed; however, you want to keep this fairly thick. Yogurts also vary by flavor. So Delicious cultured coconut is one brand that works well in this recipe. Other plain coconut yogurts can be a touch sweet, but most soy-based plain yogurts will work well.

Per ¼-cup serving: 122 calories, 4 g protein, 10 g carbohydrate, 4 g sugar, 8 g total fat, 55% calories from fat, 1 g fiber, 301 mg sodium

Balsamic Reduction

Makes ⅓ cup

Drizzle this slightly sweet syrup over homemade veggie burgers, steamed greens, pasta, pizza, soups, and more!

½ cup balsamic vinegar

2 tablespoons pure maple syrup

1 tablespoon tamari

In a saucepan, combine all the ingredients and bring to a boil over medium-high heat. Reduce the heat and simmer gently for 25 to 30 minutes. At that time, it should have thickened and become more concentrated. Let cool. It will thicken a little more with cooling.

Per 1-tablespoon serving: 42 calories, 0.4 g protein, 9 g carbohydrate, 8 g sugar, 0 g total fat, 0% calories from fat, 0 g fiber, 195 mg sodium

Cheese Replacements

"Cream Cheese"

Makes 1 cup

Use in recipes, or as a replacement for standard cream cheese to spread on bagels and sandwiches. For a variation, try the Sour Cream 'n' Onion "Cream Cheese" below.

    1 cup soaked raw cashews
    ¼ cup plain nondairy yogurt
    1 tablespoon freshly squeezed lemon juice
    1½ teaspoons pure maple syrup
    ¼ teaspoon guar gum (optional, see Note)
    ¼ teaspoon (rounded) sea salt

In a blender (see Note), blend all the ingredients until very smooth, scraping down the side of the blender as needed. Use straightaway or refrigerate in an airtight container for 3 to 5 days.

Guar Gum Note: The guar gum helps create a slight viscous texture to the cheese, which more resembles commercial cream cheese (dairy or nondairy). It's not essential to the flavor, however. So, if you don't have it, you can omit and simply chill the mix to help it set before serving.

Blender Note: This recipe works best in a high-speed blender with a small jar. If you use a large jar, double the batch; it will move in the blender much more easily for a smoother puree.

   Per 2-tablespoon serving: 98 calories, 3 g protein, 7 g carbohydrate, 2 g sugar, 7 g total fat, 62% calories from fat, 1 g fiber, 149 mg sodium

Sour Cream 'n' Onion "Cream Cheese"

Makes 1 cup

    1 cup soaked raw cashews
    ¼ cup plain nondairy yogurt
    1 tablespoon freshly squeezed lemon juice
    2 tablespoons sliced green onion (green portion)
    1 teaspoon chickpea miso or other mild miso
    ½ teaspoon pure maple syrup

⅛ teaspoon (lightly rounded) guar gum (optional, see Note)

¼ teaspoon (rounded) sea salt

In a blender (see Note), blend all the ingredients until very smooth, scraping down the side of the blender as needed. Once smooth, use straightaway or refrigerate in an airtight container for 3 to 5 days.

Guar Gum Note: The guar gum helps create a slight viscous texture to the cheese, which more resembles commercial cream cheese (dairy or nondairy). It's not essential to the flavor, however. So, if you don't have it, you can omit and simply chill the mix to help it set before serving.

Blender Note: This recipe works best in a high-speed blender with a small jar. If you use a large jar, double the batch; it will move in the blender much more easily for a smoother puree.

Per 2-tablespoon serving: 98 calories, 3 g protein, 6 g carbohydrate, 2 g sugar, 7 g total fat, 62% calories from fat, 1 g fiber, 176 mg sodium

Tofu "Feta"
Makes 2 cups (4 servings)

Tofu and Brine

1 (12-ounce) package extra-firm tofu, cut into ½- to ¾-inch cubes (see Note)

1½ cups water

¼ cup red wine vinegar

2 cloves garlic, roughly sliced or chopped

½ teaspoon sea salt

Marinade

1½ tablespoons chickpea miso or other mild miso

2 tablespoons freshly squeezed lemon juice

1½ tablespoons red wine vinegar (or 2 tablespoons for extra tang)

½ teaspoon pure maple syrup

1 teaspoon dried oregano

¼ to ⅓ cup minced green olives or kalamata olives

To brine the tofu: In a large saucepan, combine all the ingredients and bring to a boil. Reduce the heat and simmer for 15 to

20 minutes, uncovered. If some of the tofu is not covered in the brine, stir occasionally to distribute evenly

Meanwhile, to make the marinade: In a medium bowl or baking dish, combine the miso, lemon juice, vinegar, maple syrup, and oregano. Whisk well, then stir in the olives.

Strain the tofu, discarding the brine (it's okay to keep the garlic). While still hot/warm, transfer the tofu to the bowl with the marinade. Stir gently to coat the tofu and combine well (see Note). Cover and refrigerate for up to a week. The tofu will absorb the flavors as it sits.

Tofu Note: When working the marinade through the tofu it's okay if the tofu breaks up into uneven pieces rather than uniform cubes (it's quite good that way)!

Per serving (¼ of recipe): 113 calories, 9 g protein, 6 g carbohydrate, 2 g sugar, 7 g total fat, 49% calories from fat, 1 g fiber, 674 mg sodium

Soy-Free "Feta"

Makes 2 cups (4 servings)

½ cup soaked raw cashews
½ cup soaked almonds (or additional ½ cup soaked cashews)
2½ tablespoons freshly squeezed lemon juice
2 teaspoons apple cider vinegar
1½ teaspoons brine from jar of olives
1½ tablespoons chickpea miso or other mild miso (but not soy-free miso)
¾ teaspoon dried oregano
½ teaspoon sea salt
¼ cup sliced green olives (or kalamata olives, but the color of the feta will change)

Combine the cashews, almonds, lemon juice, vinegar, brine, miso, oregano, and salt in a food processor or high-powered blender (see Note) and blend until smooth. Add the olives and just pulse in.

Transfer the mixture to a sieve lined with a damp cheesecloth that has been set over a bowl to catch any drippings. Cover with plastic wrap and refrigerate overnight.

The next day, discard any liquid caught from the drippings (there may not be much), and unmold the cheese from the cheesecloth. Serve, spreading on crackers or breads, or refrigerate again until ready to use, up to one week.

Variation: For a firmer feta, use agar: Follow the directions through pulsing in the olives. Then, combine 2½ to 3 teaspoons agar powder with ⅓ to ½ cup water and heat in a small saucepan over medium-high heat. Heat until it begins to bubble and thicken, a minute or two. Use a spatula to incorporate the agar mixture into the cashew mixture, either in the blender or after transferring to a bowl. Incorporate well. Transfer the mixture to a dish that has been lightly oiled. Cover and refrigerate. After several hours the mixture will be firm enough to cut in cubes or crumble.

Blender Note: This recipe works best in a high-speed blender with a small jar. If you use a large jar, double the batch. It will move in the blender much more easily for a smoother puree. If not using a high-powered blender, double the batch for a food processor to get a good, smooth puree (it won't be as smooth as in a high-powered blender, but it will still be good).

> *Per serving (¼ of recipe):* 221 calories, 8 g protein, 12 g carbohydrate, 2 g sugar, 18 g total fat, 67% calories from fat, 3 g fiber, 672 mg sodium

Tangy Cashew "Cheese"

Makes 2½ cups

This cheese makes a beautiful spread, but can also be layered in baked pasta dishes, or paired with baked potatoes.

    2½ cups soaked raw cashews
    1 tablespoon chickpea miso or other mild miso
    2 tablespoons freshly squeezed lemon juice
    1 tablespoon apple cider vinegar or rice vinegar
    ½ teaspoon sea salt
    ½ teaspoon probiotic powder (roughly from 2 capsules; optional, see Note)
    4 to 7 tablespoons water (as needed)

In a food processor or high-speed blender, blend the cashews, miso, lemon juice, vinegar, salt, probiotic powder (if using), and 4 tablespoons water until smooth and creamy. Stop to scrape down the side of the processor/blender as needed, adding additional water to thin as desired.

If using the probiotic powder, place the cheese in a bowl and cover with plastic wrap. Let sit at room temperature for about 24 hours to allow the flavor to develop. (If not using the probiotic, simply transfer the blended mixture to the fridge until serving.) Serve, or refrigerate or freeze in portions. Keeps in fridge for up to one week.

Probiotic Note: Two probiotic brands to look for are Garden of Life Primal Defense and Natural Factors Ultimate Probiotic. The probiotic powder can be omitted and the cheese will still have a wonderful flavor.

Leftovers Note: If you have leftovers, they freeze well. Store portions in small airtight containers and freeze, then thaw at room temperature for several hours before serving.

Per 3-tablespoon serving: 137 calories, 5 g protein, 8 g carbohydrate, 2 g sugar, 11 g total fat, 65% calories from fat, 1 g fiber, 139 mg sodium

"Parmesan"

Makes 1½ cups

1½ cups raw cashews or raw almonds
1 tablespoon nutritional yeast
½ teaspoon sea salt
1½ tablespoons freshly squeezed lemon juice

Preheat the oven to 300°F. Line a baking sheet with parchment paper.

Process the nuts in a food processor or blender until fine and crumbly (don't process too long or they will get sticky). Transfer to the baking sheet and add the nutritional yeast, salt, and lemon juice. Mix all the ingredients together well on the sheet, then distribute evenly.

Bake, tossing several times during baking, until golden, about 30 minutes (check often during the last minutes, as the nuts can quickly turn from golden to too brown). Let cool on the baking sheet. Transfer to a container and refrigerate for weeks to a couple of months.

Per 3-tablespoon serving: 139 calories, 5 g protein, 8 g carbohydrate, 2 g sugar, 11 g total fat, 65% calories from fat, 1 g fiber, 149 mg sodium

Nut-Free "Parmesan"

Makes ¾ cup

½ cup unsweetened flaked coconut (or scant ½ cup unsweetened shredded coconut)
½ cup sunflower seeds
¼ cup pumpkin seeds
1½ tablespoons nutritional yeast
¼ teaspoon sea salt
1½ tablespoons freshly squeezed lemon juice

Preheat the oven to 275°F and line a baking sheet with parchment paper.

In a food processor or blender, process the coconut, sunflower seeds, and pumpkin seeds until fine and crumbly. Don't overprocess, or they will begin to heat and become pasty; just pulse until finely crumbled. Transfer to the parchment and add the nutritional yeast, salt, and lemon juice. Use your fingers to work these ingredients through, then spread evenly.

Bake, being sure to toss two or three times during the baking process, for 25 to 30 minutes; check during last minutes of baking—the mixture should be dry and maybe a touch golden around the edges, but should not be brown. Let cool and transfer to a container to store in the fridge for weeks to a couple of months.

Per 3-tablespoon serving: 224 calories, 8 g protein, 9 g carbohydrate, 1 g sugar, 19 g total fat, 72% calories from fat, 4 g fiber, 156 mg sodium

Melt-y "Mozza"

Makes ⅔ cup

1 cup water
3 tablespoons raw cashew butter
3 tablespoons tapioca starch
1½ teaspoons freshly squeezed lemon juice
1 teaspoon chickpea miso or other mild miso
½ teaspoon sea salt

In a high-speed blender (see Note), puree all ingredients until smooth. Transfer to a small saucepan, scraping out all the mix. Heat over medium or medium-low heat, whisking continuously. In about 3 minutes, the mixture will become a little curdled, and then in the next minute or two it will form into a ball. Once at this stage, remove from the heat. Use straightaway for dipping or spreading, or let cool. After cooling, scoop spoonfuls on pizza, toasts, or use to top pasta bakes. Keeps in refrigerator for up to 5 days.

Blender Note: A high-speed blender works best. If using a standard blender, scrape down the side of the jar several times.

Per 3-tablespoon serving: 112 calories, 3 g protein,
11 g carbohydrate, 1 g sugar, 7 g total fat, 51% calories from fat,
0.4 g fiber, 394 mg sodium

Tofu "Ricotta"
Makes about 2 cups

Marinade
1 tablespoon tahini
1 tablespoon freshly squeezed lemon juice
1½ teaspoons chickpea miso or other mild miso
1½ teaspoons rice vinegar
1 teaspoon pure maple syrup
½ teaspoon garlic powder
½ teaspoon (slightly rounded) sea salt

1 (14-ounce) package medium-firm tofu, pressed (see Note)
Couple pinches ground nutmeg (optional)
Minced fresh basil/parsley/chives (optional)

Make the marinade: In a large bowl, whisk together all of the marinade ingredients.

Break up the tofu with your hands and mash or mix into the marinade. Add the nutmeg and fresh herbs if using. You can keep some chunkier texture. Use a spoon to incorporate the marinade well. Let sit for 30 minutes or longer. Refrigerate for up to 2 to 3 days and use in lasagna or other pasta bakes.

Tofu Note: Use a medium-firm tofu in this recipe, rather than firm or extra-firm. The texture is softer and smoother for a ricotta replacement. It's very useful to press the tofu as well. Use a tofu press, draining the liquid a few times over an hour. If you don't have a tofu press, wrap the tofu in one or two layers of paper towel, and then with a tea towel. Place between two plates or cutting boards, and weigh down (with a heavy pot or books). Press for a half hour or longer, and drain off all liquid.

Per 5-tablespoon serving: 63 calories, 5 g protein, 3 g carbohydrate, 1 g sugar, 4 g total fat, 52% calories from fat, 0.5 g fiber, 355 mg sodium

Herbed "Cheese" Ball
Serves 6

Cheese Ball

1½ cups soaked raw cashews

1 tablespoon nutritional yeast

1 tablespoon chickpea miso or other mild miso

2 teaspoons apple cider vinegar or rice vinegar

1½ teaspoons white wine (see Note)

½ teaspoon Dijon mustard

½ teaspoon sea salt

1 small clove garlic, sliced

1½ teaspoons fresh thyme leaves (see Note)

1 tablespoon chopped fresh chives or green portion of green onion (optional)

Coating

3 tablespoons chopped raw or toasted nuts (such as pistachios or walnuts)

1 tablespoon minced fresh chives or green portion of green onion

2 tablespoons dried cranberries or Coconut Bacon (page 232)

To make the cheese ball: In a food processor, combine all the ingredients except the thyme and chives and process until the mixture becomes smooth. Add the thyme and chives and pulse a couple of times to lightly incorporate. Transfer to a container, cover, and refrigerate for about an hour.

Combine the coating ingredients on a sheet of parchment. Form the cheese into a ball with your hands (lightly oil your hands to make it easier), and then gently roll the ball around the parchment to pick up the coating. Return to the fridge in a covered container until ready to use. Keeps refrigerated for up to a week.

Wine Note: If you don't have white wine, substitute another 1 teaspoon vinegar and ½ teaspoon apple or orange juice, or 1½ teaspoons seasoned rice vinegar.

Herb Note: If you don't have fresh thyme, don't substitute dried. Instead, substitute another leafy herb, such as 3 to 4 tablespoons torn/chopped fresh basil leaves, or 1 to 2 tablespoons fresh chopped parsley, or just use the green onion/chives.

Per serving (⅙ of recipe): 222 calories, 8 g protein, 15 g carbohydrate, 4 g sugar, 16 g total fat, 61% calories from fat, 2 g fiber, 316 mg sodium

Smoky Tomato–Almond "Cheese" Ball
Serves 6

2 cups soaked almonds
⅓ cup sun-dried tomatoes (see Note)
3 tablespoons freshly squeezed lemon juice
2 tablespoons chickpea miso or other mild miso
1½ tablespoons natural ketchup
2 teaspoons smoked paprika
1 teaspoon fresh rosemary leaves
½ teaspoon garlic powder
½ teaspoon sea salt

Coating

3 tablespoons finely chopped raw or toasted almonds
    (or other nuts)
1 to 2 tablespoons chopped fresh chives
Pinch sea salt

To make the cheese ball: In a food processor, pulse the almonds until crumbly. Add the remaining cheese ball ingredients and process until the mixture becomes sticky and forms a mound on the blade. (If mixture isn't coming together, add a teaspoon or two of water, as the almonds may be dry.) Transfer to a container and refrigerate for about an hour.

Combine the coating ingredients on a sheet of parchment. Form the cheese mixture into a ball with your hands (lightly oil your hands to make it easier), and gently roll around the parchment to pick up the coating. Return to the fridge in a covered container until ready to use. Keep in fridge for up to one week.

Sun-Dried Tomato Note: If using packaged sun-dried tomatoes that are dry, reconstitute in a bowl of boiled water for 5 to 10 minutes, then drain and pat dry.

Per serving (⅙ of recipe): 327 calories, 12 g protein, 17 g carbohydrate, 5 g sugar, 26 g total fat, 67% calories from fat, 8 g fiber, 559 mg sodium

Snacks and Dips

Greek Chickpeas

Makes about 1¾ cups (3 servings)

These roasted chickpeas are delicious all on their own—and so nibbly you may want to double or triple the batch! You can also add them to salads, pack into lunches, or sprinkle on pizza. Or lightly puree a handful in a mini–food processor with tahini and a few seasonings for a chunky spread for sandwiches.

   1 (15-ounce) can chickpeas, rinsed and drained

   3 tablespoons chopped kalamata olives

   2 tablespoons brine from jarred olives

   ½ to ¾ teaspoon chopped fresh rosemary

   ½ teaspoon pure maple syrup

   ¼ teaspoon sea salt

Preheat the oven to 450°F. Line a baking sheet with parchment paper.

   On the baking sheet, combine all the ingredients and toss to combine. Roast for 20 to 25 minutes, until the chickpeas are a light golden and the marinade is absorbed. Serve warm.

   Per serving (⅓ of recipe): 139 calories, 6 g protein, 22 g carbohydrate, 4 g sugar, 3 g total fat, 21% calories from fat, 6 g fiber, 489 mg sodium

Easy, Creamy Hummus

Makes generous 4 cups

   2 (15-ounce) cans chickpeas, rinsed and drained

   1 (15-ounce) can white beans, rinsed and drained

   ⅓ cup freshly squeezed lemon juice

   2 tablespoons tahini

   1 tablespoon chopped fresh parsley

   1 medium clove garlic, peeled

   ½ teaspoon smoked paprika, plus more to taste

   ½ teaspoon ground cumin

1¼ teaspoons sea salt

Several cubes of ice and/or few tablespoons of cold water, to thin as desired

In a food processor, combine all the ingredients except the ice. Puree, and when starting to become smooth, add the ice or water to help smooth out. Use just enough to get it smooth but still with a thick texture. Taste, and add up to ¼ teaspoon additional smoked paprika or other seasonings to taste.

Per ½-cup serving: 171 calories, 9 g protein, 26 g carbohydrate, 3 g sugar, 4 g total fat, 20% calories from fat, 7 g fiber, 571 mg sodium

Roasted Tomato and Garlic Chickpea Dip

Makes 4 cups

Serve this zesty dip room temp with whole-grain crackers, breads, or tortilla chips. Or use in wraps or spread on pizza.

1½ pounds roma (or other) tomatoes, cut in half and juices gently squeezed out (see Note)

8 to 9 large cloves garlic, peeled and cut into quarters or smaller

2 tablespoons balsamic vinegar

1½ teaspoons tamari (or coconut aminos for soy-free option)

1 teaspoon blackstrap molasses

2 teaspoons dried oregano

2 teaspoons dried basil

⅛ teaspoon plus ¾ teaspoon sea salt

Freshly ground black pepper

2 (15-ounce) cans chickpeas, drained and rinsed

2 tablespoons tahini

Preheat the oven to 450°F.

Place the tomatoes cut side up in a glass baking dish (or a small rimmed baking sheet lined with parchment paper). Insert the garlic pieces into the seedy portions of the tomatoes (to keep them moist while roasting). In a small bowl, combine the balsamic, tamari, molasses, oregano, and basil and drizzle over the tomatoes. Sprinkle with the ⅛ teaspoon salt and with pepper to taste. Roast for 40 to 45 minutes, until the tomatoes are very soft and a little caramelized. Let cool.

Meanwhile, combine the chickpeas, tahini, and ¾ teaspoon salt in a food processor and puree to break up.

Add the tomatoes to the processor, scraping in all the juices with a spatula. Process until well combined. Taste, and if you'd like extra salt (or pepper), add and puree again.

Tomato Note: Roma tomatoes work well here as they are dense and meaty, with less seeds than other tomatoes. But other beautifully ripe tomatoes can be substituted!

Per ½-cup serving: 141 calories, 6 g protein, 21 g carbohydrate, 5 g sugar, 4 g total fat, 24% calories from fat, 5 g fiber, 477 mg sodium

Nacho Dip

Makes 4½ cups (5 servings)

Serve with tortilla chips, or to top potatoes or beans, or as part of a Mexican platter. If you like, add some veggies to the dip, just before adding the salsa. Try chopped bell peppers, pitted olives, sliced green onions, chopped baby spinach, or corn kernels. Or add a cup or so of black beans.

2 cups plain unsweetened nondairy milk

1 cup soaked raw cashews

½ cup frozen cubed sweet potato or cooked sweet potato

¼ cup potato flour, or 1 cup cooked potato

2 tablespoons freshly squeezed lemon juice

1 tablespoon apple cider vinegar

1 tablespoon tahini

2 teaspoons chickpea miso or other mild miso

1 small clove garlic, peeled and cut into small pieces

¼ teaspoon smoked paprika

1¼ teaspoons sea salt

¾ to 1 cup mild salsa, to taste (use medium spicy for extra heat)

Preheat the oven to 400°F. Grease an 8 x 8-inch baking dish (or similar) by wiping or spraying the inner surface with a touch of oil.

In a blender, combine all ingredients except the salsa and puree until very smooth. Transfer to the prepared dish. Add the salsa, and just swirl it slightly into the dip (if you have children who don't like salsa, swirl into just a portion of the dip). Bake for 25 minutes, until thickened and bubbly. Let cool for 5 minutes.

Per serving (⅛ of recipe): 255 calories, 10 g protein, 25 g carbohydrate, 6 g sugar, 15 g total fat, 49% calories from fat, 4 g fiber, 991 mg sodium

Salads and Sides

Sesame Quinoa Salad
Makes scant 3 cups (2 main-dish servings)

2 cups cooled cooked quinoa

½ cup thawed frozen green peas or steamed sliced snow peas

½ cup grated carrot (standard grate, not fine) or store-bought shredded carrot

¼ cup diced red bell pepper

1 tablespoon chopped green onion (green portion)

1 to 2 tablespoons toasted sesame seeds, for garnish (optional)

Dressing

3 tablespoons rice vinegar

1½ tablespoons tahini

2 tablespoons tamari (or coconut aminos)

1½ tablespoons pure maple syrup

½ to 1 teaspoon grated fresh ginger (use Microplane grater)

¼ teaspoon garlic powder

In a large bowl, combine the quinoa, peas, carrot, red pepper, and green onion.

To make the dressing: In a separate bowl, whisk together the ingredients until the tahini is fully incorporated.

Add the dressing to the quinoa mixture, and mix to combine well. Serve, sprinkling with the toasted sesame seeds, if using.

Per serving (½ of recipe): 389 calories, 14 g protein, 61 g carbohydrate, 17 g sugar, 10 g total fat, 22% calories from fat, 8 g fiber, 1072 mg sodium

Mango and Salsa Bean Salad
Makes 6 cups (5 servings)

1 to 1½ cups cubed fresh mango (1 medium mango) (see Note)

1 cup diced red bell pepper

1 (15-ounce) can black beans, rinsed and drained

1 (15-ounce) can pinto beans, rinsed and drained
¼ cup salsa, or more if desired
2 to 3 tablespoons sliced chives or green onion
2 to 2½ tablespoons freshly squeezed lime juice
1 teaspoon pure maple syrup
½ teaspoon ground cumin
⅛ teaspoon ground allspice
½ teaspoon sea salt, plus more to taste (see Note)
2 to 3 tablespoons minced cilantro (optional)

In a large bowl, combine all the ingredients and stir. Taste, and if you'd like more heat and zip from the salsa, add a little more, up to another ¼ cup. Serve, or refrigerate (covered) for several hours until ready to serve.

Mango Note: If not serving right away, reserve the mango and add just before serving. This will preserve its freshness and flavor.

Salt Note: The amount of salt you use may depend on the brand of salsa. Start with ½ teaspoon, as it's always easy to add extra later.

Per serving (⅕ of recipe): 186 calories, 10 g protein, 36 g carbohydrate, 8 g sugar, 1 g total fat, 5% calories from fat, 11 g fiber, 562 mg sodium

Oil-Free Croutons

Makes 3 cups (4 servings)

1 clove garlic, peeled and halved (optional)
1½ tablespoons aquafaba (see Note)
¼ teaspoon onion powder or garlic powder
¼ teaspoon paprika or smoked paprika
¼ teaspoon sea salt
3 cups 1-inch-cubed whole-grain bread
1½ teaspoons Balsamic Reduction (page 215, or see Note)
   (optional)

Preheat the oven to 400°F. Line a baking sheet with parchment paper. If using the garlic, rub it generously around inside of a large bowl (this will infuse a garlic flavor that isn't too intense). Discard the clove or save for another use.

Add the aquafaba to the bowl and whisk in the onion powder, paprika, and salt. Coat the inner surface of the bowl with the aquafaba mixture, then add the cubed bread and immediately toss to coat the cubes as evenly as possible.

Transfer to the parchment-lined baking sheet and bake for 10 to 12 minutes, stirring once during baking time. Check at around 10 minutes, and if the croutons look golden and are becoming crisp, remove (they will crisp more as they cool). If not, let them bake for another minute or two, checking in on them frequently, as they can turn from golden to burned very quickly. If using the Balsamic Reduction, drizzle over the croutons. Let cool on pan until ready to use.

Aquafaba Note: A fancy word for "bean water," aquafaba is simply the liquid drained from a can of beans, preferably white beans or chickpeas. This bean water has been found to be useful as an egg replacer, and here it helps the seasonings adhere to the croutons without the use of oil.

Balsamic Reduction Note: Instead of making your own balsamic reduction, you can try one of the balsamic reductions available in stores. They are usually with the salad dressings or in the deli section with the specialty oils and spreads.

> *Per serving (¼ of recipe):* 76 calories, 4 g protein, 13 g carbohydrate, 1 g sugar, 1 g total fat, 13% calories from fat, 2 g fiber, 282 mg sodium

Coconut Bacon

Makes 2 cups

The flavor surpasses store-bought varieties; it's worth a little effort to make! Sprinkle it on finished pizzas, soups, or salads, or try it in sandwiches with avocado and veggies.

1 tablespoon coconut sugar

2½ tablespoons tamari

1½ teaspoons balsamic vinegar

½ teaspoon liquid smoke (see Note)

¾ teaspoon smoked paprika

¼ teaspoon garlic powder
½ teaspoon (scant) sea salt
Freshly ground black pepper, to taste
2 cups large flaked, unsweetened coconut

Preheat the oven to 275°F. Line a baking sheet with parchment paper.

In a large bowl, combine the coconut sugar, tamari, balsamic, liquid smoke, paprika, garlic powder, salt, and black pepper. Mix until the sugar is dissolved. Add the coconut and mix until all the marinade is absorbed and the coconut is fully coated.

Spread on the prepared baking sheet and bake for 30 to 32 minutes, tossing once about halfway during baking, until dark pinkish brown. Be sure to check for doneness early—at 27 or 28 minutes—as the coconut can turn from just perfectly cooked to burned (dark brown, and with a bitter flavor) in just a few minutes. So, don't overbake! Let cool. The bacon will continue to dry and crisp once out of the oven. Once completely cool, transfer to an airtight container and refrigerate; it will keep for weeks, maybe longer!

Liquid Smoke Note: While this is not an ingredient you may use often, it has a unique and essential flavor. It is worth adding to your kitchen (it stores well in the fridge). You can find it in many grocery stores and also specialty/health food stores. It is not a chemical product; rather, it's made from condensing vapors from the smoke of smoldering wood chips.

Per ¼-cup serving: 141 calories, 2 g protein, 7 g carbohydrate, 3 g sugar, 13 g total fat, 77% calories from fat, 3 g fiber, 439 mg sodium

Rosemary Sweet Potato Fries

Serves 5 as a side

2 tablespoons freshly squeezed lemon juice
1 tablespoon pure maple syrup
1½ teaspoons Dijon mustard
1 to 1½ teaspoons minced fresh rosemary leaves, to taste
½ teaspoon onion powder
3 pounds yellow sweet potatoes, peeled and cut into wedges
½ teaspoon sea salt

Preheat the oven to 400°F. Line a large, rimmed baking sheet with parchment paper and spray the parchment lightly with oil (or wipe a little over with a paper towel).

In a large bowl, whisk together the lemon juice, maple syrup, mustard, rosemary, and onion powder. Add the sweet potato wedges and mix to coat. Transfer the potatoes to the prepared baking sheet and pour over any remaining liquid. Sprinkle with the salt.

Bake for 55 to 65 minutes (or longer), rotating and flipping the wedges once or twice, until the sweet potatoes have softened and are caramelized (delicious!) in spots.

Per serving (⅙ of recipe): 163 calories, 3 g protein, 38 g carbohydrate, 13 g sugar, 0.5 g total fat, 2% calories from fat, 6 g fiber, 330 mg sodium

Bruschetta

Serves 4 as a side (or more as an appetizer)

Sliced crusty bread (see Note)
1½ cups chopped seeded tomatoes (or sliced grape/cherry tomatoes, seeds squeezed out)
¼ cup chopped kalamata olives
¼ cup sliced green onions (mostly green portion)
1½ teaspoons balsamic vinegar
½ teaspoon dried oregano
1 small clove garlic, grated (or ¼ teaspoon garlic powder)
¼ teaspoon (scant) sea salt
½ cup Tofu "Feta" (page 217), crumbled (optional)

Preheat the oven to 400°F. Line a baking sheet with parchment paper.

Place the bread slices on the parchment. Bake for 8 to 9 minutes, until golden. Let cool slightly.

Meanwhile, in a bowl, combine the remaining ingredients and stir thoroughly.

Place spoonfuls of the tomato mixture on each slice of bread. Return to the oven and bake for 10 to 12 minutes, until edges of bread are crispy and golden, and toppings are lightly heated through.

Bread Note: How much sliced bread you need depends on the type of bread and the size of the slices. A full baguette could be used here, or about half of a larger artisanal loaf of bread.

Per serving (¼ of recipe, topping only): 27 calories, 1 g protein, 4 g carbohydrate, 2 g sugar, 1 g total fat, 33% calories from fat, 1 g fiber, 184 mg sodium

Soups and Stews

Cream of Broccoli Soup
Serves 4

1 to 2 tablespoons water
1½ cups chopped onion
1 teaspoon dry mustard
½ teaspoon dill seed (don't substitute dill weed)
¾ teaspoon sea salt
Freshly ground black pepper, to taste
4 cups roughly chopped broccoli (florets and trimmed stems)
½ cup soaked raw cashews
1½ cups plain nondairy milk, or more to thin the soup
½ cup water
2 tablespoons freshly squeezed lemon juice
1½ teaspoons chickpea miso or other mild miso
Pinch nutmeg
¼ cup fresh basil leaves (optional, but very good)

In a large pot, combine 1 tablespoon water, the onion, mustard, dill seed, salt, and pepper. Cook over medium-high heat for 8 to 9 minutes, stirring occasionally, until onions have softened; add a touch more water if the onions are sticking. Add the broccoli, reduce the heat to medium-low, cover, and cook for 4 to 5 minutes, until broccoli turns bright green. Don't let the broccoli overcook; keep it a vibrant green color. Remove from the heat.

Meanwhile, puree the cashews and 1 cup of the milk in a blender until smooth. Add the remaining ½ cup milk, the ½ cup water, lemon juice, miso, and nutmeg and puree again.

Transfer the sautéed onion and broccoli to the blender, along with the basil if using. Puree until fairly smooth (you can smooth as much as you like). Taste, and add extra salt and pepper as desired, and additional nondairy milk or water to thin if needed.

Per serving (¼ of recipe): 179 calories, 9 g protein,
19 g carbohydrate, 5 g sugar, 9 g total fat, 44% calories
from fat, 5 g fiber, 596 mg sodium

Curried Carrot and Sweet Potato Soup
Serves 4

2 tablespoons water

1 to 1¼ cups chopped onion

2 cups chopped carrots

3 cups chopped orange sweet potatoes

1 tablespoon grated fresh ginger

1½ teaspoons curry powder

½ teaspoon ground cinnamon

Few pinches freshly grated nutmeg

1¼ teaspoons sea salt

4 cups water

1 dried bay leaf

2 to 3 tablespoons coconut milk (see Note) or Luscious Cashew
    Cream (page 212) (optional)

1½ tablespoons freshly squeezed lemon juice

Heat the 2 tablespoons water in a large pot over medium or medium-high heat. Add the onion, carrots, sweet potatoes, ginger, curry powder, cinnamon, nutmeg, and salt. Stir, cover, and cook, stirring occasionally, for 8 to 9 minutes until onions soften. Add the 4 cups water and the bay leaf and bring the mixture to a boil. Lower the heat to medium-low, cover, and simmer for 25 minutes.

Remove and discard the bay leaf. Use an immersion blender to puree the soup. (Or, transfer the soup to a high-speed blender and puree, but you will need to let the soup cool some before blending and puree in a couple of batches.) Add the coconut milk (if using) and lemon juice. Puree the soup until completely smooth. Season to taste and serve.

Coconut Milk Note: Use full-fat coconut milk from a can. It's optional, but adds great texture.

Per serving (¼ of recipe): 134 calories, 3 g protein, 28 g carbohydrate, 10 g sugar, 2 g total fat, 13% calories from fat, 6 g fiber, 805 mg sodium

Mushroom Chili

Serves 6

1½ cups diced onion
1½ tablespoons balsamic vinegar
1 tablespoon mild chili powder
2 teaspoons dried oregano
1 teaspoon smoked paprika
¼ teaspoon ground cinnamon or allspice
½ teaspoon crushed red pepper flakes, or to taste
1 teaspoon sea salt, plus more to taste
1 to 1½ pounds white mushrooms, roughly chopped (7 to 8 cups)
4 to 5 cloves garlic, minced
1 cup diced green or red bell pepper
1 (28-ounce) can or 1 (26-ounce) box low-sodium crushed tomatoes
1 (15-ounce) can pinto beans or kidney beans, rinsed and drained
½ cup dried red lentils, rinsed and drained
½ cup water
½ to 1 teaspoon pure maple syrup
Freshly ground black pepper, to taste
1 cup frozen corn kernels (or more cooked beans)
Lime wedges, for serving
Hot sauce, for serving (optional)

In large pot over medium heat, combine the onion, vinegar, chili powder, oregano, paprika, cinnamon, pepper flakes, and salt. Cook, stirring occasionally, for 4 to 5 minutes, until spices are very fragrant and onions are starting to soften. Add the mushrooms and cook for 5 to 7 minutes, until they release their juices and begin to reduce. Do not add water; let the juices release from the mushrooms.

Add the garlic and bell pepper, reduce the heat, and stir for a couple of minutes. Add the tomatoes, beans, lentils, and water and stir to combine. Increase the heat and bring to a boil. Reduce the heat to low, cover, and simmer for 30 minutes, until lentils are fully cooked through and almost dissolved. Taste, and add maple syrup to taste and/or extra salt and pepper to balance flavor as desired. Stir in the corn. Let sit for a few minutes until the corn has warmed through. Serve with lime wedges and hot sauce, if desired.

Per serving (⅙ of recipe): 199 calories, 11 g protein, 39 g carbohydrate, 9 g sugar, 2 g total fat, 7% calories from fat, 10 g fiber, 549 mg sodium

African Peanut, Bean, and Vegetable Stew

Serves 6

2 to 3 tablespoons water
1 cup chopped onion
1 cup sliced fresh carrots (or frozen sliced carrots)
1½ cups chopped red or yellow bell pepper
2 to 3 large cloves garlic, minced
1½ teaspoons ground cumin
1 teaspoon ground coriander
1 teaspoon dried basil
1 teaspoon ground ginger
½ teaspoon ground cinnamon
¼ teaspoon crushed red pepper flakes, or more to taste
1¼ teaspoons sea salt
2½ to 3 cups water
1½ cups cubed sweet potatoes (or frozen sweet potatoes)
1 (15-ounce) can chickpeas, rinsed and drained
1 (15-ounce) can black beans, rinsed and drained
3 tablespoons peanut butter (or almond or cashew butter), or more to taste (see Note)
2 tablespoons freshly squeezed lime juice
Lime wedges, for serving
Chopped fresh cilantro, for serving (optional)

In a large pot, combine the 2 tablespoons water, onion, carrots, bell pepper, garlic, cumin, coriander, basil, ginger, cinnamon, pepper flakes, and salt. Cover and cook for 5 to 7 minutes, stirring once or twice, until vegetables are starting to soften. If sticking, add another splash of water.

Add the 2½ cups of water, sweet potatoes, chickpeas, beans, and peanut butter and stir to combine. Increase the heat and bring to a boil. Reduce the heat to low, cover, and simmer for 10 to 15 minutes or longer, until the sweet potatoes and carrots have softened. (With 2½ cups of water, this soup remains fairly thick. Feel free to thin out with another ½ cup of water or more.)

Stir in the lime juice and taste. Season if desired with additional lime juice or salt. Serve with lime wedges and fresh cilantro if using.

Peanut Butter Note: If you want a richer broth in the stew, use an additional 1 tablespoon peanut butter.

Add-Ins: Add spinach for color: Just before serving, while the soup is hot, stir in a few cups baby spinach leaves until just wilted.

Per serving (⅙ of recipe): 236 calories, 10 g protein, 38 g carbohydrate, 8 g sugar, 6 g total fat, 22% calories from fat, 11 g fiber, 737 mg sodium

Lentil and Split Pea Soup with Fennel and Orange
Serves 6 or more

2 to 3 tablespoons water
1½ cups diced onion
2 cups chopped fennel bulb (about 1 large bulb)
1 cup chopped parsnip
1 cup chopped carrots
1 teaspoon ground ginger
1 teaspoon paprika
1 teaspoon dried oregano
1 teaspoon dried rosemary
½ to 1 teaspoon fennel seed
1¼ teaspoons sea salt, plus more to taste
1 cup dried yellow split peas, rinsed and drained
1 cup dried red lentils, rinsed and drained
5 cups water
2 dried bay leaves
½ cup freshly squeezed orange juice
Freshly ground black pepper, to taste

In a large soup pot over medium heat, combine 2 tablespoons water, the onion, fennel, parsnip, carrots, ginger, paprika, oregano, rosemary, fennel seed, and salt and stir to combine. Cover and cook for 8 to 10 minutes, until onions soften; stir occasionally and add an extra splash of water if sticking.

Add the split peas and lentils to the pot along with the 5 cups water and bay leaves. Stir to combine. Increase the heat and bring to a boil. Reduce the heat to low, cover, and simmer for 50 to 60 minutes (or a little longer), until the split peas and lentils are completely softened. Remove and discard the bay leaves. Stir in the orange juice and season with additional salt and pepper if desired.

Per serving (⅙ of recipe): 258 calories, 16 g protein, 49 g carbohydrate, 7 g sugar, 1 g total fat, 3% calories from fat, 17 g fiber, 529 mg sodium

Pasta, Pizza, Burgers, and Other Mains

Luscious Fettuccine Alfredo
Serves 4

1 (1-pound) package whole-wheat fettuccine (or other dry pasta)
½ cup soaked raw cashews
1 tablespoon tahini
2 teaspoons chickpea miso or other mild miso
2 to 3 cloves garlic, peeled
½ teaspoon dry mustard
1 teaspoon sea salt
1½ cups plain nondairy milk
½ cup cooked peeled red or yellow potato (roughly cubed or
    crumbled to measure)
1½ tablespoons freshly squeezed lemon juice
Few pinches freshly grated nutmeg and/or black pepper
¼ to ⅓ cup water

Cook the pasta in a large pot of salted boiling water according to package directions. Drain and return to the pot.

Meanwhile, in a blender, puree the cashews, tahini, miso, garlic, mustard, salt, and 1 cup of the milk until very smooth. Add the remaining ½ cup milk, the potato, juice, and nutmeg and puree until smooth. Makes about 2½ cups sauce.

Transfer the sauce to the pasta pot. Use the water to swish and "rinse" all the sauce from the blender, and add to the pasta. Gently heat the pasta with the sauce over medium-low heat, tossing, until the sauce thickens, just a minute or two. Serve.

Per serving (¼ of recipe): 535 calories, 23 g protein,
91 g carbohydrate, 4 g sugar, 13 g total fat, 20% calories from fat,
11 g fiber, 741 mg sodium

Sweet Potato–Tahini Sauce

Makes 2½ cups (5 servings)

1 cup cooked peeled orange or yellow sweet potato (broken apart
    to measure)

⅓ cup tahini

1 tablespoon freshly squeezed lime juice or rice vinegar

1 tablespoon pure maple syrup

½ to 1 tablespoon roughly chopped peeled fresh ginger (see
    Note)

2 small or medium cloves garlic, peeled (see Note)

⅛ teaspoon crushed red pepper flakes (optional, see Note)

¾ teaspoon sea salt

1 cup water, plus more if needed

Cooked rice, quinoa, millet, or other cooked grain, for serving (or
    cooked pasta such as soba noodles)

Lime wedges, for serving

In a blender, or with an immersion blender in a deep cup, puree the
sweet potato, tahini, lime juice, maple syrup, ginger, garlic, pepper
flakes (if using), salt, and 1 cup water. (The sauce will thicken
with refrigeration, and again if heating through with pasta or other
noodles. So, use 1 cup to begin, then add another few tablespoons
to thin as needed at time of serving.)

To serve, gently heat the sauce in a saucepan, then spoon over
rice or quinoa or mix into hot pasta. Serve with lime wedges to
squeeze a pop of extra zing on individual servings.

Note: If you'll be serving the sauce to children, use the lesser amount
of garlic and ginger, and then adjust to taste after. Similarly, you may
want to omit the red pepper flakes for kids.

Per ½-cup serving (sauce only): 140 calories, 4 g protein,
14 g carbohydrate, 5 g sugar, 9 g total fat, 52% calories from fat,
3 g fiber, 385 mg sodium

Pumpkin Lentil Curry
Serves 5

This curry has lots of spice flavor but not spice heat. If you'd like some heat, add ¼ teaspoon or more crushed red pepper flakes or a spicier curry powder along with the other spices when sautéing the onions.

2 to 3 tablespoons water

1 cup finely chopped onion

1 tablespoon mild curry powder

1 teaspoon ground coriander

½ teaspoon ground cinnamon

½ teaspoon garam masala

1 teaspoon sea salt

1½ cups dried green or brown lentils, rinsed and drained

1 (15-ounce) can pumpkin puree or sweet potato puree

2¾ cups water

2 cups chopped apples

1½ to 2 tablespoons freshly squeezed lemon juice (optional, but perks up flavor nicely)

Luscious Cashew Cream (page 212), for serving (to drizzle on finished portions)

In a large pot, combine 2 tablespoons water, the onion, curry powder, coriander, cinnamon, garam masala, and salt. Cover and cook over medium or medium-high heat, stirring once, for 4 to 5 minutes, until onion starts to soften. If the onion sticks, add another splash of water.

Add the lentils and stir for a few minutes, then add the pumpkin and the water. Increase the heat to high and bring to a boil. Reduce the heat to low, add the apples, cover, and simmer for 45 to 50 minutes (or longer), until the lentils are tender and the water is absorbed. If the curry is too liquid for your taste, you can reduce it (uncovered) for another 15 minutes or so. Add the lemon juice, stir to incorporate, and serve with a drizzle of cashew cream.

Per serving (⅕ of recipe, without cashew cream): 257 calories, 16 g protein, 50 g carbohydrate, 10 g sugar, 1 g total fat, 4% calories from fat, 14 g fiber, 483 mg sodium

Chickpea Tacos

Makes 5 cups taco filling (4 servings)

Serve this mildly spicy (or not!) taco filling in taco shells with Avocado Cream (page 212), rich Sour Cream (page 214), lettuce, and other fresh veggies like chopped tomatoes, jicama, or cucumber. Or serve the filling simply over rice with the toppings, or tuck all into a whole-grain tortilla.

    2 (15-ounce) cans chickpeas, rinsed and drained
    2 tablespoons water, plus more if needed
    ¾ cup chopped onion
    1 cup minced zucchini and/or bell pepper
    2 teaspoons chili powder
    2 teaspoons ground cumin
    2 teaspoons smoked paprika
    1 teaspoon garlic powder
    1 teaspoon dried oregano
    ¼ teaspoon allspice
    ¼ teaspoon crushed red pepper flakes (or fresh minced chile
        pepper to taste, see Note)
    ¾ teaspoon sea salt
    3 tablespoons freshly squeezed lime juice
    1 teaspoon molasses

Mash the chickpeas by pressing with the bottom of a measuring cup on a cutting board. (This doesn't have to be thorough, just a rough mash/squish of most of the beans.)

Heat the water in a skillet over medium-high heat. Add the onion, zucchini and/or bell pepper, chili powder, cumin, paprika, garlic powder, oregano, allspice, pepper flakes, and salt. Cook, stirring occasionally, for 6 to 8 minutes, until the onion has softened. If the mixture is drying out and sticking, add another splash of water. Add the mashed chickpeas, lime juice, and molasses and stir thoroughly. Reduce the heat to medium and cook, stirring, for 8 to 10 minutes, until mixture is heated through. Taste, and if you'd like extra salt or heat, add additional seasonings. If mixture is still dry or sticking, add another 2 to 3 teaspoons of water, increase the heat briefly, and scrape the skillet to help bring up the spices from the bottom.

Chile Pepper Note: If you'd prefer adding some chopped jalapeño or other hot pepper to this mixture instead of crushed red pepper flakes—go for it! Add as much as you normally like.

Per serving (¼ of recipe, filling only): 228 calories, 11 g protein, 39 g carbohydrate, 9 g sugar, 5 g total fat, 17% calories from fat, 11 g fiber, 773 mg sodium

Mac 'n' Trees

Serves 6

1 to 1¼ pounds dry whole-grain cut pasta (such as macaroni, penne, fusilli)

2 cups unsweetened plain nondairy milk

1 cup water

1⅓ cups soaked raw cashews

½ cup frozen cubed sweet potato or cooked sweet potato (see Note)

3½ tablespoons freshly squeezed lemon juice

2 tablespoons tahini

1 tablespoon chickpea miso or other mild miso

½ teaspoon garlic powder (not garlic salt)

½ teaspoon sea salt

¼ teaspoon black salt (see Note, page 210) (optional)

3 cups broccoli florets or cauliflower florets

1 cup dried whole-grain breadcrumbs

Preheat the oven to 400°F. Grease a 9 x 12-inch, 2½-inch-deep (or larger) baking dish by wiping the inside surface with a smidgen of oil.

Cook the pasta in a large pot of salted boiling water according to package directions until a couple minutes short of al dente.

Meanwhile, in a blender, combine the milk, water, cashews, sweet potato, lemon juice, tahini, miso, garlic powder, sea salt, and black salt (if using) and blend until very smooth.

Once the pasta is nearing al dente stage, add the broccoli and cook for just a minute, until the broccoli has just turned a bright green and the pasta is al dente but still not fully tender (as it will absorb some liquid as it bakes). Drain, but do not rinse.

Pour about one-third of the sauce in the prepared dish. Add all of the pasta and broccoli, then pour the remaining sauce over the top, distributing evenly. If needed, gently mix to incorporate the sauce. Mix the breadcrumbs with a pinch sea salt in a small bowl, then sprinkle over the top of the casserole.

Cover with foil and bake for 17 to 18 minutes. Remove the foil and bake 10 to 12 minutes longer, until the topping is golden brown and crisped. Let sit for a few minutes. Taste, season as desired, and serve.

Sweet Potato Note: If you don't have sweet potato, a good substitute is frozen sliced carrots or frozen cubed squash. Fresh carrots can also be used, if lightly steamed.

Per serving (⅙ of recipe): 529 calories, 22 g protein, 78 g carbohydrate, 7 g sugar, 18 g total fat, 29% calories from fat, 10 g fiber, 454 mg sodium

Whole-Grain Pizza

Makes 1 pizza crust (3 servings)

Along with the Pizza Sauce (page 248), top our parbaked crust with your choice of grilled or roasted vegetables (bell peppers, eggplant, zucchini), sliced grape tomatoes, sliced green onions, pitted olives, capers, sliced cooked potato or sweet potato, pineapple, artichokes, roasted garlic cloves, chickpeas (or Greek Chickpeas, page 226), and Melt-y "Mozza" (page 221). Or, instead of a tomato sauce base, try using a spread of Pistachio Pesto (page 250), hummus, or Tangy Cashew "Cheese" (page 219).

1 cup (scant) warm water (see Note)
2¼ teaspoons (1 packet) quick-rising yeast
1½ teaspoons coconut sugar
1¼ cups whole-grain spelt flour
1 cup oat flour
3 tablespoons ground flax seed (flax meal)
½ teaspoon sea salt

Combine the warm water, yeast, and sugar in a small bowl. Whisk well, then let stand for 5 to 8 minutes, until foamy.

In a large bowl, combine the spelt flour, oat flour, flax, and salt and mix well. Once the yeast mixture is foamy, add it to the flour and use a large spoon to work the mixture together. Lightly oil another bowl (large enough to hold double the size of dough), and add the dough. Cover with plastic wrap, place in a warm spot, and let rise for 1 to 2 hours, until dough has expanded up to double its original size.

If using a pizza stone, place it in the oven. Preheat the oven to 450°F.

Transfer the dough to a lightly floured work surface and knead just a few times. Shape into a ball. If not using straightaway, refrigerate for a few hours, until ready to use.

Lightly spray a large piece of parchment or wipe the surface with oil (just a very light coat to prevent sticking). Transfer the dough to the parchment, and press out with your fingers to shape into an 11- to 12-inch round. No need to make perfectly round, it looks even better with a rustic shape! Use a pizza peel or large plate to transfer the dough (on the parchment) to the pizza stone or a baking sheet. Bake for 8 to 9 minutes (see Note). Add toppings of choice (see ideas on page 247), then return to the oven until the toppings are heated through and the crust is golden brown, about 6 to 10 minutes.

Warm Water Note: The water should be warm to the touch—not hot, as that will kill the yeast, but not too cold, as that will not activate it.

Baking Note: Parbaking the dough helps prevent a soggy crust in the middle, especially if piling on the veggies! So, bake for 8 to 9 minutes, then remove, add toppings, and finish baking. You can even allow the crust to cool in advance before adding toppings.

Per serving (⅓ of recipe, crust only): 374 calories, 15 g protein, 67 g carbohydrate, 5 g sugar, 7 g total fat, 16% calories from fat, 12 g fiber, 403 mg sodium

Pizza Sauce

Makes generous 1½ cups sauce (enough for at least 2 large pizzas)

¾ cup water
1 (6-ounce) can tomato paste (about ¾ cup)
2 tablespoons pure maple syrup

1½ teaspoons balsamic vinegar
1½ teaspoons dried basil
1 teaspoon dried oregano
½ to 1 teaspoon garlic powder (see Note)
½ teaspoon sea salt, plus more to taste
Freshly ground black pepper, to taste

Combine all the ingredients in a bowl and whisk to mix. Season to taste with extra salt and pepper if desired. Refrigerate if not using right away, or spread on pizza crusts as thin/thick as you like.

Seasoning Suggestions: The seasonings used here add a base flavor without being too spicy or overpowering. If you want to add more flavor, use the full 1 teaspoon garlic powder (or add freshly minced or grated garlic or roasted garlic), or add onion powder, lemon pepper, smoked paprika, chopped fresh rosemary/oregano/basil, chopped chives, or crushed red pepper flakes.

Per ¼-cup serving: 44 calories, 1 g protein, 10 g carbohydrate, 8 g sugar, 0.2 g total fat, 3% calories from fat, 1 g fiber, 421 mg sodium

So-Simple Lentil Pasta Sauce

Makes 4½ cups (5 servings)

Toss this robust sauce with whole-grain pasta (a 1-pound package works well) for a hearty dinner. Also use as a sauce to layer in lasagna, or in burritos or to top a cooked grain.

1½ cups water
½ cup dried green or brown lentils, rinsed and drained
5 cloves garlic, peeled and scored or squished (but not chopped, to infuse flavor)
½ to 1 tablespoon balsamic vinegar (see Note)
Pinch or two sea salt (to taste, see Note)
1 (16-ounce or similar size) jar pasta sauce (see Note)

In a medium or large pot, combine the water, lentils, and garlic and bring to a boil over high heat. Reduce the heat to low, cover, and cook for 35 to 40 minutes, until the lentils are fully tender. Remove the garlic cloves, or leave in for more flavor (see Note).

Add the vinegar, salt, and pasta sauce and gently heat through over medium-low heat. Taste, adding additional seasonings if you like.

Balsamic Note: We enjoy a punch of flavor from balsamic vinegar in pasta sauces. You can taste this sauce without it first, and then add a small amount, and taste to see if you like it, then add more to taste.

Salt Note: Jarred pasta sauces vary in flavor, and also in salt content. So, you may want to adjust the salt to your taste. Start with a pinch or two, and add more as needed.

Sauce Note: Opt for a store-bought pasta sauce that is lower in sweeteners, oil, and salt (those ingredients should be listed toward the end of ingredient list, rather than near the beginning). Organic varieties tend to have more natural and healthful ingredients.

Garlic Note: If you leave the garlic in, you can keep the cloves whole, or use the back of a spoon to squish and work into the sauce.

> *Per serving (⅛ of recipe):* 151 calories, 7 g protein,
> 27 g carbohydrate, 11 g sugar, 3 g total fat, 17% calories from fat,
> 5 g fiber, 549 mg sodium

Pistachio Pesto

Makes about 1½ cups (4 servings)

Toss this bright, vibrant green sauce with 1 pound of whole-grain pasta (such as Kamut pasta, brown rice pasta, or whole-wheat pasta), using as much pesto as desired, and adding extra water to help thin and coat the pasta. Squeeze on some fresh lemon juice and serve. Or keep the pesto thick, and it will work beautifully as a spread for sandwiches or pizza, or to dollop on potatoes or soup.

1 cup raw pistachios
1 tablespoon tahini
¼ cup freshly squeezed lemon juice (zest first, see Note), plus more to taste
1 large clove garlic, peeled
½ to 1 teaspoon sea salt (see Note)
3 cups loosely packed fresh basil leaves
¼ cup fresh parsley (optional, for color, but nice!)

2 to 4 tablespoons water, as needed

½ teaspoon grated lemon zest

In a blender or food processor, combine the pistachios, tahini, lemon juice, garlic, and salt and begin to pulse/puree to break up, scraping down the side of the bowl as needed. Add the basil and parsley and puree until fairly smooth (or leave some texture). You will need some water to get it smooth; start with 2 tablespoons, and see if that's enough. If you need more, add a little at a time. Stir in the lemon zest. Store in an airtight container in refrigerator until ready to use. Keeps for 3 to 4 days.

Lemon Zest Note: Be sure to zest the lemon before juicing it (as it is difficult to zest a juiced lemon). A kitchen rasp (Microplane grater) works really well for zesting.

Salt Note: You can adjust the salt based on how you plan to use the pesto. If you like a lot of pesto on your pasta, ½ teaspoon salt may be enough. If spreading the same amount of pesto over more pasta, you may need the full teaspoon for seasoning. So, start with ½ teaspoon and adjust to taste. Also, if using this pesto as a spread for bread or pizza, the salt will be more concentrated and you may want to use less.

Per serving (¼ of recipe, sauce only): 204 calories, 8 g protein, 11 g carbohydrate, 3 g sugar, 16 g total fat, 66% calories from fat, 4 g fiber, 298 mg sodium

Spinach–Sweet Potato Lasagna

Serves 6

5 cups good-quality low-sodium pasta sauce, about
1½ (26-ounce) jars

1 (12-ounce) package whole-grain ready-bake lasagna noodles
(see Note)

Tofu "Ricotta" (page 222)

4 to 5 cups baby spinach, roughly torn

1½ to 2 cups cooked sweet potatoes, roughly mashed with a
pinch of salt and pepper (see Note)

¼ cup sliced kalamata olives (optional)

3 tablespoons "Parmesan" (page 220), or ⅓ cup Tangy Cashew
"Cheese" (page 219), or sprinkle of commercial grated vegan
cheese

Preheat the oven to 375°F. Lightly oil a roughly 9 x 13-inch lasagna casserole dish.

Spread 1 cup of the pasta sauce over the bottom of the dish. Cover with 3 or 4 noodles (depending on size). Next, spread roughly half of the ricotta and roughly half of the spinach over the noodles. Arrange 3 or 4 noodles in the opposite direction on top. Layer on the sweet potatoes and olives (if using), plus 1½ cups sauce. Top with another 3 or 4 noodles in the opposite direction, then the remainder of the ricotta and spinach. Add the remaining noodles, again in the opposite direction to previous layer, and top with the remaining 2½ cups of sauce. Sprinkle on the Parmesan or dollop on the cashew cheese (or sprinkle/crumble on commercial cheese).

Cover the dish tightly with foil and bake for 55 to 60 minutes, until the noodles are fully cooked when pierced through. Let rest for 10 minutes before slicing and serving.

Noodle Note: Using ready-bake noodles makes lasagna prep a lot easier, although you do need to use a little extra sauce to soften the noodles. If you'd like to use standard lasagna noodles, parboil the noodles first, cooking until not fully done, and use about 6 cups sauce total.

Sweet Potato Note: You can substitute different veggies for the sweet potatoes, such as roasted veggies, artichoke hearts, grilled sliced mushrooms, or sliced cooked yellow potatoes.

Per serving (⅙ of recipe): 450 calories, 19 g protein, 77 g carbohydrate, 19 g sugar, 10 g total fat, 19% calories from fat, 11 g fiber, 536 mg sodium

Italian "Meatballs"

Makes about 20 balls (4 servings)

Serve these irresistible meatless balls with whole-grain pasta and your favorite store-bought tomato sauce.

¼ cup chopped sun-dried tomatoes (if they are tough, cut with kitchen shears)

1 medium clove garlic, peeled

1 cup lightly toasted walnuts (or toasted pecans or toasted
  pumpkin seeds)

1 cup rolled oats

1 teaspoon dried oregano

½ teaspoon dried basil

½ teaspoon fennel seeds

½ teaspoon sea salt

1 teaspoon balsamic vinegar

½ to 1 teaspoon vegan Worcestershire sauce

1 cup (broken up or cubed) cooked peeled red or Yukon gold
  potatoes

Preheat the oven to 375°F. Line a baking sheet with parchment
paper.

In a food processor, combine the sun-dried tomatoes and garlic
and pulse to break up. Add the walnuts, oats, oregano, basil, fennel
seeds, and salt and process until very crumbly. Add the balsamic
and Worcestershire and pulse the mixture a couple of times. Finally,
add the potato. Puree briefly, until the mixture just comes together.
(Pureeing the potato too long can make the meatballs gummy.)

Scoop about 1-tablespoon portions of the mixture, form into balls,
and place on the baking sheet. Bake for 17 to 20 minutes, until lightly
browned (do not overbake, they will dry out).

Variations: For burgers, form the mixture into patties and bake for
9 to 10 minutes on each side. Have leftovers? Use as filling for
a lunch wrap or crumble on pizza. Or, make Italian meatball
sandwiches with Melt-y "Mozza" (page 221) and your favorite pasta
sauce.

Per serving (¼ of recipe, about 5 meatballs): 287 calories,
8 g protein, 28 g carbohydrate, 3 g sugar, 18 g total fat,
52% calories from fat, 5 g fiber, 374 mg sodium

Salsa Bean Burgers

Makes 10 patties

Instead of serving on buns, try serving these zesty patties in crispy romaine leaves.

2 (15-ounce) cans kidney beans, rinsed, excess water drained, and beans patted dry with a paper towel

⅓ cup mild salsa (see Note)

1 tablespoon tahini

1 medium clove garlic, sliced or quartered

1 teaspoon smoked paprika

1 teaspoon dried oregano

1½ teaspoons cumin

½ teaspoon grated lime zest (optional)

½ teaspoon (rounded) sea salt

½ cup sliced green onions (mostly green portions)

3 to 4 tablespoons chopped cilantro leaves (optional)

1¼ cups rolled oats

½ to ¾ cup frozen corn

Sliced avocado, Avocado Cream (page 212), or Sour Cream (page 214), for serving (optional)

Preheat the oven to 400°F. Line a baking sheet with parchment paper.

In a food processor, combine the beans, salsa, tahini, garlic, paprika, oregano, cumin, lime zest (if using), and salt. Puree until well combined. Add the green onions, cilantro (if using), and oats and pulse a couple of times to break up and combine. Remove the blade and stir in the corn. Shape the mixture into 10 patties. (You can refrigerate mixture for about a half hour before shaping, but that's not essential.)

Place the patties on the baking sheet and bake for 8 to 10 minutes on one side, then flip and bake another 8 to 10 minutes on the second side, until the patties have become a little golden and more firm. Or, cook in a nonstick skillet over medium heat for 6 to 8 minutes on each side, until golden brown. Serve topped with avocado, Avocado Cream, or Sour Cream if you like.

Salsa Note: A mild salsa keeps the flavors family-friendly. For extra heat, use a medium or hot salsa. Textures of salsa can vary, and watery salsa will make these burgers loose, so you may want to drain the salsa first: To get the ⅓ cup, measure out ½ cup and drain in a sieve so only the chunkier parts remain.

> *Per serving (¹⁄₁₀ of recipe, patties only):* 132 calories, 7 g protein, 23 g carbohydrate, 3 g sugar, 2 g total fat, 14% calories from fat, 5 g fiber, 360 mg sodium

Omega Burgers

Makes 8 patties

1 cup cooled cooked dark orange squash (such as red kuri or kabocha) or cooked peeled sweet potatoes (see Note)

2 tablespoons natural ketchup

1 teaspoon apple cider vinegar

1 tablespoon nutritional yeast (optional)

1 teaspoon Dijon mustard

1 teaspoon garlic powder

1 teaspoon onion powder

1 teaspoon dried basil

1 teaspoon sea salt

2 cups (lightly packed) cooled cooked brown rice

½ cup rolled oats

½ cup hemp seeds

½ cup pumpkin seeds (see Note)

1 tablespoon ground chia seeds

In a large bowl, roughly mash the squash, mixing in the ketchup, vinegar, nutritional yeast, mustard, garlic powder, onion powder, basil, and salt. Add the rice, oats, hemp seeds, pumpkin seeds, and chia seeds and mix to fully incorporate. Transfer the bowl to the fridge and chill for 30 minutes or longer.

Preheat the oven to 400°F. Line a baking dish with parchment.

Shape the mixture into 8 patties. Place the patties in the dish and bake for 9 to 10 minutes on one side, then flip and bake for another 9 to 10 minutes on the second side, until the patties have become a little golden and more firm. Serve warm.

Squash Note: The easiest way to cook squash or sweet potatoes is to bake whole, without cutting or piercing. Place whole squash or potatoes on a baking sheet lined with parchment paper and bake at 425°F for 40 to 60 minutes, until soft (cooking time will depend on size of squash/sweet potato).

Pumpkin Seed Note: If you prefer the texture, you can opt to pulse the pumpkin seeds in a food processor before adding to burgers.

> *Per serving (⅛ of recipe):* 191 calories, 7 g protein,
> 23 g carbohydrate, 2 g sugar, 8 g total fat, 38% calories from fat,
> 6 g fiber, 348 mg sodium

Marinated Mushroom Burgers

Serves 3 (2 caps per person)

Serve with whole-grain buns and all the fixin's!

6 medium or large portobello mushrooms
2½ tablespoons balsamic vinegar
1½ teaspoons pure maple syrup
1½ teaspoons vegan Worcestershire sauce
1 teaspoon garlic powder
½ teaspoon onion powder
Sea salt and freshly ground black pepper, to taste

Preheat a grill to high or medium-high.

Using a damp towel or paper towel, wipe the mushroom caps to gently clean. Use a spoon to scrape the gills from the underside of the mushrooms. Discard the scrapings.

In a large bowl, combine the vinegar, maple syrup, Worcestershire sauce, garlic powder, and onion powder, whisking well. Add the mushroom caps and gently turn in the marinade to coat evenly.

Place the mushrooms (scraped side up) on the grill and sprinkle on a pinch of salt and pepper. Grill for 5 to 7 minutes on the first side, until grill marks have formed and the mushrooms have softened slightly. Flip, and cook for another 3 to 4 minutes, until the caps are cooked through.

> *Per serving (⅓ of recipe without bun):* 59 calories, 4 g protein,
> 11 g carbohydrate, 7 g sugar, 1 g total fat, 9% calories from fat,
> 3 g fiber, 45 mg sodium

Desserts

Vanilla Bean Chocolate Cake

Makes two 9-inch cakes (10 servings)

Serve this decadent chocolate cake with the Dreamy Chocolate Frosting on page 258.

2 cups whole-grain spelt flour

½ cup coconut sugar

⅓ cup cocoa powder

2 teaspoons baking soda

¾ teaspoon vanilla bean powder, or 2 teaspoons pure vanilla extract (if using extract, add with wet ingredients)

¼ teaspoon (rounded) sea salt

3 tablespoons coconut butter, softened (see Note)

½ cup pure maple syrup, at room temperature

1½ cups water, at room temperature

2 tablespoons rice vinegar or apple cider vinegar

2 tablespoons nondairy mini or regular chocolate chips (optional)

Preheat the oven to 350°F. Grease two 9-inch round cake pans by lightly wiping with oil (or spraying with oil); place a round of parchment paper on the bottom of each pan.

In a large bowl, mix the flour, sugar, cocoa, baking soda, vanilla powder, and salt. In a separate bowl, combine the coconut butter with the maple syrup (and vanilla extract if using), mixing to combine well. Add the water and vinegar and mix again. Add the wet mixture to the dry, and stir in the chocolate chips (if using) just until well combined.

Pour the batter into the prepared pans and bake for 22 to 24 minutes, until golden and a toothpick or skewer inserted in the center comes out clean. Let cool fully on a cooling rack before frosting.

Coconut Butter Note: To soften coconut butter, place measured amount in a small ovenproof bowl. Place in a warm (not hot) oven (around 250°F). Check after about 5 minutes, and once softened enough so you can easily stir, remove from oven. Alternatively, you can place in a dish in a hot water bath and stir the mix occasionally until the heat from the hot water bath gradually melts/softens the coconut butter. It's important to have the water and maple syrup at room temperature so that the coconut butter doesn't seize up when mixing.

Per serving (⅒ of recipe): 197 calories, 4 g protein, 40 g carbohydrate, 22 g sugar, 4 g total fat, 16% calories from fat, 4 g fiber, 376 mg sodium

Dreamy Chocolate Frosting

Makes 2¼ cups

This will modestly frost a two-layer cake. For a very thick layer of frosting on a two-layer cake, double the batch. This is divine on the Vanilla Bean Chocolate Cake (page 257)!

1 (12-ounce) package extra-firm silken tofu, patted dry (see Note)
1 to 2 tablespoons pure maple syrup (see Note)
½ teaspoon pure vanilla extract
Pinch sea salt
1¼ cups nondairy chocolate chips

In a blender or food processor (not a mixer, it won't smooth the tofu), combine the tofu with 1 tablespoon maple syrup, the vanilla and salt, and puree until very, very smooth, scraping down the side of the bowl as needed.

Meanwhile, melt the chocolate in a bowl fitted over a pot (or the top of a double boiler) with simmering water. Pour the melted chocolate into the tofu mixture and puree again until smooth (again, scraping down the side of the bowl). Taste, and add the extra maple syrup if you like, and puree again. Transfer to a container and refrigerate (it will thicken as it cools).

Tofu Note: Be sure to use silken tofu here, not standard tofu (they have completely different textures). Choose the extra-firm silken.

Maple Syrup Note: For me, this frosting is sweet enough with just 1 tablespoon maple syrup, but depending on the brand of chocolate chips, you may want to add more syrup to sweeten the frosting for the kiddos.

Per serving (¹⁄₁₀ of recipe): 123 calories, 3 g protein,
14 g carbohydrate, 12 g sugar, 7 g total fat, 50% calories
from fat, 1 g fiber, 44 mg sodium

Chocolate–Peanut Butter Gelato

Makes 2 cups (4 servings)

½ cup cold coconut cream (from can of regular coconut milk,
    see Note)
1 cup (lightly packed) pitted dates (see Note)
¾ cup sliced overripe frozen banana
⅓ cup cocoa powder
1 to 2 tablespoons pure maple syrup (optional, see Note)
¼ teaspoon sea salt
2 tablespoons peanut butter (or almond or cashew butter), or
    more to taste

In a food processor or high-speed blender, puree the coconut
cream and dates until the dates break down. Add the banana,
cocoa powder, 1 tablespoon maple syrup (if using), and salt. Puree
until very smooth. This mixture will be very thick, so you will need to
scrape down the blender/processor a few times. Taste, and if you'd
like a touch more sweetness, add an additional 1 tablespoon maple
syrup.

Transfer to a container, then drop in the peanut butter in spots.
Use a knife or spoon to lightly swirl or cut the peanut butter through
the mixture. Taste, and swirl in additional peanut butter if you want
more richness. Transfer to the freezer and freeze for 4 to 5 hours, until
frozen but still easy to scoop. You can also serve after just 2 to
3 hours of freezing; it will be like a soft-serve.

Coconut Milk Note: Use the cream that rises to the top of a 14-ounce
can of regular coconut milk (rather than light coconut milk). Be sure
to first refrigerate overnight (or a few days) so the thick cream will rise
to the top and be easy to scoop and measure. Use only the thick
cream. You can also use the cream from a small (5.5-ounce) can. It
won't be quite ½ cup, but will be close enough!

Date Note: Dates must be soft to easily puree. Some pitted dates can be old and dry. If your dates aren't soft, try soaking them in nondairy milk for a half hour or so until they soften.

Maple Syrup Note: This ice cream is naturally sweet with the dates, so you may omit the maple syrup if you generally don't like things too sweet. If not using the syrup, substitute more coconut cream or some nondairy milk to help with the blending.

Per ½-cup serving: 292 calories, 5 g protein, 42 g carbohydrate, 29 g sugar, 16 g total fat, 45% calories from fat, 7 g fiber, 184 mg sodium

Caramel Banana Ice Cream
Makes 2½ cups (4 servings)

1 small (5.5-ounce) can regular coconut milk (not reduced-fat)
½ cup pitted dates (see Note)
¼ cup coconut sugar
¼ teaspoon vanilla bean powder (or ½ teaspoon pure vanilla extract)
Couple pinches grated nutmeg
⅛ teaspoon sea salt
2 cups frozen sliced overripe bananas (see Note)

In a blender, puree the coconut milk with the dates until the dates are mostly smoothed out. Add the sugar, vanilla, nutmeg, and salt and puree again to incorporate. Add 1 cup of the banana and pulse in. Add the remaining banana and pulse/puree until fully smooth. Once smooth, you can serve, though it may be slightly loose. If so, transfer to a container to freeze for an hour or more. Once firmer, scoop and serve!

Date Note: If your dates aren't very soft, first soak them in water for an hour or so, until softened, then fully drain.

Frozen Banana Note: You can freeze overripe bananas in batches when you have them. Peel, then slice and store in a Ziploc bag. You can keep them in the freezer for months, ready to use.

Per ½-cup serving: 200 calories, 2 g protein, 37 g carbohydrate, 28 g sugar, 7 g total fat, 29% calories from fat, 3 g fiber, 63 mg sodium

Chocolate Almond Macaroons

Makes 18 cookies

1 cup unsweetened shredded coconut

1 cup almond meal

⅓ cup cocoa powder

1 teaspoon baking powder

¼ teaspoon sea salt

⅓ cup brown rice syrup

¼ cup pure maple syrup

1 teaspoon pure vanilla extract

3 tablespoons nondairy chocolate chips (optional)

Preheat the oven to 350°F. Line a baking sheet with parchment paper.

In a bowl, combine the coconut, almond meal, cocoa, baking powder, and salt and mix until well combined. In another bowl, stir together the rice syrup, maple syrup, and vanilla. Add the wet mixture and the chocolate chips (if using) to the dry mixture and mix until combined.

Use a small cookie scoop (or spoon) to scoop 1-tablespoon portions of batter onto the prepared baking sheet. (If you have a very large sheet, place all cookies on one sheet with just a little room between each; for a smaller sheet, bake in two batches.) Bake for 14 minutes, until set to the touch (they will still be a little soft inside). Let cool on the baking sheet for a minute, then transfer to a cooling rack to cool completely.

Per cookie: 105 calories, 2 g protein, 12 g carbohydrate, 5 g sugar, 7 g total fat, 53% calories from fat, 2 g fiber, 71 mg sodium

No-Bake Iced Gingerbread Bars
Makes 20 squares

Bars
1½ cups plus 2 tablespoons rolled oats

⅓ cup almond meal (or unsweetened shredded coconut for nut-
   free bars)

1½ teaspoons ground cinnamon

½ to 1 teaspoon ground ginger (use 1 teaspoon for more punch)

¼ teaspoon sea salt

2 cups (lightly packed) pitted dates

¼ cup raisins

1 teaspoon pure vanilla extract (or ¼ teaspoon vanilla powder)

Icing
½ cup (loosely packed) coconut butter (not oil)

3 tablespoons pure maple syrup

2½ tablespoons nondairy milk

Couple pinches sea salt

¼ to ½ teaspoon grated lemon zest (optional)

Line a 8 x 8-inch baking pan with parchment paper.

To make the bars: In a food processor, combine the oats, almond meal, cinnamon, ginger, and salt and pulse a few times to get the oats crumbly. Add the dates, raisins, and vanilla and pulse a few times to start to incorporate. Then, begin to puree steadily, and continue until the mixture becomes cohesive (it will form a large ball on the blade). Remove the dough, and press it evenly into the prepared pan.

To prepare the icing: Combine the coconut butter, maple syrup, milk, and salt and gently warm. You can do this in a bowl set over a hot water bath or in an ovenproof bowl in the oven/toaster oven at low heat—see the Note on page 257 for how to soften coconut butter. (Be careful not to scorch the coconut butter, just warm it until it softens.) Once softened, mix until smooth and add the lemon zest if using.

Pour the icing over the dough, and spread to distribute evenly (or leave it a little more rustic if you like). Chill in the refrigerator for a couple of hours and then cut into bars.

Per bar: 130 calories, 2 g protein, 21 g carbohydrate, 13 g sugar, 5 g total fat, 33% calories from fat, 3 g fiber, 63 mg sodium

Divine Cheesecake
Serves 8

Crust

1½ cups rolled oats
¼ cup almond meal
1 cup pitted dates
½ teaspoon pure vanilla extract
⅛ teaspoon sea salt

Filling

1½ cups soaked raw cashews
1 cup coconut butter (not oil)
⅓ cup plain or vanilla nondairy yogurt (or unsweetened applesauce)
⅓ cup pure maple syrup
¼ cup freshly squeezed lemon juice
½ teaspoon grated lemon zest (optional)
½ teaspoon guar gum (optional, see Note)
¼ teaspoon (scant) sea salt
Lightly oil a 9-inch springform pan.

To make the crust: Combine all the ingredients in a food processor. Pulse to get moving, and then process until the mixture becomes quite sticky and holds together when pressed between your fingers. Transfer to a springform pan and press onto the bottom of the pan (not up the sides).

To make the filling: Combine all the ingredients in a blender (high-powered blender is best). Puree until very, very smooth (stopping to scrape down the blender a couple of times as needed).

Pour the filling over the crust and tip the pan back and forth to evenly distribute. Cover the pan with foil and pop in freezer until set, 3 to 4 hours or overnight.

To serve, soften at room temperature for about a half hour. Slice, and serve as is or with Raspberry Dessert Sauce (below).

Guar Gum Note: This cheesecake can be made without the guar gum. Guar gum is a plant-based thickener that helps stabilize blends like puddings, creams, ice creams, etc. It lends more viscosity to the final texture, but isn't critical. So, it's fine if you don't have it on hand.

Per serving (⅛ of cake): 498 calories, 10 g protein, 51 g carbohydrate, 25 g sugar, 32 g total fat, 53% calories from fat, 9 g fiber, 113 mg sodium

Raspberry Dessert Sauce

Makes about 1½ cups

3 cups fresh or frozen raspberries (see Note)
3 to 4 tablespoons pure maple syrup
½ teaspoon pure vanilla extract
Few pinches sea salt

Combine the berries, 3 tablespoons maple syrup, vanilla, and salt in a saucepan over medium heat. Bring to a slow boil, then reduce the heat to medium-low and simmer for 15 to 20 minutes, until the raspberries have softened and sauce has thickened slightly. Taste, and add additional maple syrup if desired. Serve the sauce warm or cool (it will thicken more after cooling).

Berry Note: If you'd like to substitute other berries like blueberries or chopped strawberries, go for it!

Per 3-tablespoon serving: 44 calories, 0.5 g protein, 10 g carbohydrate, 7 g sugar, 0.5 g total fat, 6% calories from fat, 3 g fiber, 111 mg sodium

Baked Bananas

Serves 3

This recipe can serve up to four if you pair with a nondairy yogurt or ice cream. Also try topping with a sprinkle of chopped toasted pecans or almonds.

4 large (or 5 small) ripe bananas, sliced lengthwise
1½ teaspoons freshly squeezed lemon juice
1 tablespoon coconut sugar
½ teaspoon ground cinnamon
Pinch sea salt

Preheat the oven to 450°F. Line a baking sheet with parchment paper.

Place the bananas on the parchment and drizzle on the lemon juice. Turn the bananas to coat in the juice. Sprinkle with the sugar, cinnamon, and salt.

Bake for 10 minutes, until the bananas are softened and caramelized. Serve warm and enjoy.

Per serving (⅓ of recipe): 179 calories, 2 g protein, 46 g carbohydrate, 26 g sugar, 1 g total fat, 3% calories from fat, 5 g fiber, 100 mg sodium

Dessert Cashew Cream

Makes about 1 cup

This easy-to-make cream is very versatile, perfect for desserts but also beautiful for special breakfasts. For instance, dollop atop Baked Bananas (above) or Lemon-Berry Pancakes (page 204), or layer with summer berries and kiwi in parfait glasses.

1 cup soaked raw cashews
⅓ to ½ cup water (plus extra to thin if desired)
2 to 3 tablespoons pure maple syrup
¼ teaspoon vanilla bean powder (see Note)
⅛ teaspoon sea salt

In a blender, or with an immersion blender in a deep cup, puree all the ingredients (starting with ⅓ cup of water and 2 tablespoons maple syrup) until smooth. If needed, add the extra water to get the mixture moving and even smoother. Taste, add extra maple syrup to sweeten or more water to thin if desired. Serve, or refrigerate until ready to use (will keep up to 5 days).

Vanilla Note: If you don't have vanilla bean powder, you can use ½ teaspoon vanilla extract, or substitute other essences to tailor to your dessert. For instance, try ½ teaspoon grated organic orange or lemon zest, or ¼ teaspoon almond extract.

> *Per 3-tablespoon serving:* 154 calories, 4 g protein, 12 g carbohydrate, 6 g sugar, 11 g total fat, 58% calories from fat, 1 g fiber, 59 mg sodium

Vanilla Whipped Cream

Makes scant 1 cup (4 servings)

1 (14-ounce) can regular (not light) coconut milk
1 to 2 tablespoons natural powdered sugar, to taste
½ teaspoon vanilla bean powder (see Note)
¼ teaspoon xanthan gum (optional, but helps stabilize)

Refrigerate the coconut milk until very cold, preferably overnight. This will help the thick cream solidify and separate from the watery liquid.

Open the can and use a spoon to scoop out the thick cream into a stand mixer. You will get just over ½ cup; if you get extra, that's fine. Use only the cream, discard the watery liquid.

Add the remaining ingredients, and with the wire whip attachment, whip the cream at high speed for a couple of minutes, until it becomes fluffy and thick. Once thickened, serve, or transfer to an airtight container and refrigerate for up to 2 or 3 days.

Vanilla Note: If you don't have vanilla bean powder, you can substitute ½ teaspoon of a good-quality vanilla extract or the seeds scraped from one vanilla bean.

> *Per serving (¼ of recipe):* 108 calories, 1 g protein, 4 g carbohydrate, 3 g sugar, 10 g total fat, 81% calories from fat, 1 g fiber, 1 mg sodium

An Elimination Diet for Identifying Problem Foods

Many people find that joint pain, headaches, and inflammatory conditions improve when they avoid certain trigger foods. But which foods are they? A food that might be tolerated perfectly well by one person might cause a massive headache for someone else.

An elimination diet will help you identify your problem foods. It is just a temporary diet change, not a permanent one, that will help you pinpoint exactly which foods work best for you. For a short period of time—ten days or so—the diet focuses on foods that are known to be safe for virtually everyone, while eliminating everything else. Then, if the pain has improved, the eliminated foods are returned to the diet in a systematic way to show whether they trigger pain. Then, in the future, you can avoid the foods that trigger your pain. Many people have long-lasting relief.

The Elimination Phase: Using Pain-Safe Foods

The elimination phase is limited to very few pain-safe foods and is not intended for long-term use. During this time, the diet emphasizes grains and cooked vegetables, with more modest portions of other foods.

Below are the pain-safe foods. Be sure to prepare abundant quantities. There are no limits on calories or portion sizes.

Grains

See the preparation tips for oatmeal and rice on page 271.

Oatmeal (unflavored)
Rice hot breakfast cereal
Brown rice (other types of rice are fine, too)
Quinoa
Rice pasta
Buckwheat
Amaranth
Millet
Teff

Vegetables

The following vegetables should be cooked until soft, generally by steaming or boiling. A standard serving would be approximately 1½ cups. Carrots can also be juiced.

Carrots
Broccoli
Brussels sprouts
Kale

Cabbage

Cauliflower

Chard

Collards

Lettuce

Squash (summer squash
   or winter squash)

Spinach

Asparagus

Fruits

Pears

Apricots

Blueberries

Plums

Legumes

Green beans

Lentils

Sweetener

Brown rice syrup

Oil

While it's best to minimize the use of oils, the addition of a modest amount of olive oil during the elimination phase is fine, either for sautéing or as a topping.

Condiments and Spices

For this short period, it is good to omit condiments and spices, other than salt.

Calories and Protein in Common Foods

In case you were wondering if you would get adequate protein during an elimination diet, here are some examples of common foods, showing their calorie and protein content. The serving sizes for cooked grains and vegetables (1½ cups) are appropriate during the diet phase that excludes many other foods, but are larger than most people would have during a more usual diet that includes many other foods.

	Calories	Protein (grams)
Old-fashioned oatmeal (1½ cups, cooked)	225	7
Rice cereal (1½ cups, cooked)	300	6
Brown rice (1½ cups, cooked)	328	7
Quinoa (1½ cups, cooked)	333	12
Broccoli or Brussels sprouts (1½ cups, cooked)	82	6
Carrots (1½ cups, cooked)	82	2
Lentils (½ cup, cooked)	115	9
Pear (1, raw)	103	1
Blueberries (½ cup, raw)	42	1

For reference, most people need about 50 grams of protein per day. A day's menu including 6 cups cooked grains, 6 cups cooked green vegetables, ½ cup lentils, and a piece of fruit, with no added oil, provides approximately 1,800 calories and 62 grams of protein.

A Word about Vitamin B_{12}

Unfortified foods from plant sources do not provide vitamin B_{12}. Over a week or two, this presents no problem, but for longer periods, vitamin B_{12} must be supplemented in the form of a vitamin supplement or fortified foods.

Making Perfect Oatmeal

Oatmeal is a handy breakfast staple during an elimination diet. If you've never cooked oatmeal, don't be afraid of the "old-fashioned" variety. The truth is, it cooks in just a few minutes, almost as quickly as instant oatmeal. Mix one part oatmeal with two parts water, bring it to a boil, then simmer for several minutes. If you like it crunchier and less creamy, boil the water before stirring in the oatmeal.

You'll find that you can vary the creaminess of other breakfast grains (e.g., rice cereal) using the same technique. If you like it creamy, add the grain to the water *before* turning on the heat. If you prefer a crunchier texture, boil the water before adding the grain.

Making Perfect Brown Rice

Brown rice is another wonderfully healthful staple. But many people find that their best efforts at cooking brown rice yield something suspiciously like wet newspaper. Here's a better way:

Start with organic short-grain brown rice. All health food stores have it. Put 1 cup rice into a saucepan and rinse it briefly with water, then drain away the water completely. You are now left with damp rice in a pan. Put the pan on high heat and stir it dry, about 1 or 2 minutes. This imparts a lovely toasted flavor.

Then add 3 cups water and bring to a boil. Reduce the heat and simmer until it is thoroughly cooked, but still retains just a hint of crunchiness—40 minutes or so. (Do not cook it until all the water is absorbed.) Then simply drain off the extra water—it will be the best brown rice you've ever tasted.

The Reintroduction Phase

If an elimination diet has eliminated or greatly reduced your pain, the next step is to nail down which foods are your triggers. To do this, simply reintroduce each eliminated food one at a time, every two days, to see whether pain results. It is important to introduce only one food at a time—that way, if pain occurs, you will have identified the culprit. Do not start by reintroducing foods you crave. Rather, start with the foods that you feel are *least* likely to cause problems. Foods that you strongly suspect to be triggers should be introduced last.

As you bring in each new food, have a generous amount, so you will know whether or not it causes symptoms. If it causes no problem, you can keep it in your diet. Anything that causes pain should be eliminated again. Later on, you may wish to try the suspect food once again for confirmation. Keep your diet simple so you can detect the effect of each newly added food. Meats, dairy products, and eggs are best left off your plate permanently.

Common Pain Triggers

The following foods have been reported to be pain triggers. Those at the top of the list are common triggers; those near the bottom are much less likely to cause problems.

    Dairy products
    Meat
    Eggs
    Chocolate
    Citrus fruits (oranges, grapefruit, lemons, limes, and citric acid)
    Corn
    Wheat, barley, and rye

Nuts and peanuts
Potatoes
Sweet potatoes
Tomatoes
Eggplant
Onions
Celery
Corn
Apples
Bananas
Alcoholic beverages
Sugar
Garbanzo beans (chickpeas)
Soy products
Coffee (both regular and caffeine-free)

Coffee can be a double-edged sword. Although some people find that the caffeine in coffee can sometimes knock out a headache that is just starting, the coffee itself seems to trigger headaches. That is, there may be some constituent of the coffee bean (other than caffeine) that acts as a pain trigger.

References

Chapter 1. The Ultimate Processed Food

1. ConsoGlobe. Planétoscope. *Statistiques mondiales en temps réelles*. Internet: http://www.planetoscope.com/elevage-viande/1044-production-mondiale-de-fromage.html. Accessed March 27, 2016.

Chapter 2. More Calories Than Coke, More Salt Than Potato Chips: What Cheese Does to Your Waistline

1. Benatar JR, Jones E, White H, Stewart RA. A randomized trial evaluating the effects of change in dairy food consumption on cardio-metabolic risk factors. *Eur J Prev Cardiol*. 2014;21(11):1376–86.

2. Benatar JR, Sidhu K, Stewart RA. Effects of high and low fat dairy food on cardio-metabolic risk factors: a meta-analysis of randomized studies. *PLoS One*. 2013;8(10):e76480.

3. Smith JD, Hou T, Ludwig DS, Rimm EB, Willett W, Hu FB, Mozaffarian D. Changes in intake of protein foods, carbohydrate amount and quality, and long-term weight change: results from 3 prospective cohorts. *Am J Clin Nutr*. 2015;101(6):1216–24.

4. Sparks LM, Xie H, Koza RA, et al. A high-fat diet coordinately downregulates genes required for mitochondrial oxidative phosphorylation in skeletal muscle. *Diabetes*. 2005;54:1926–33.

5. Hirabara SM, Curi R, Maechler P. Saturated fatty acid-induced insulin resistance is associated with mitochondrial dysfunction in skeletal muscle cells. *J Cell Physiol*. 2010;222:187–94.

6. Anderson AS, Haynie KR, McMillan RP, et al. Early skeletal muscle adaptations to short-term high-fat diet in humans before changes in insulin sensitivity. *Obesity.* 2015;23:720–24.

7. Benatar JR, Sidhu K, Stewart RA. Effects of high and low fat dairy food on cardio-metabolic risk factors: a meta-analysis of randomized studies. *PLoS One.* 2013;8(10):e76480.

8. Neves AL, Coelho J, Couto L, Leite-Moreira A, Roncon-Albuquerque R Jr. Metabolic endotoxemia: a molecular link between obesity and cardiovascular risk. *J Mol Endocrinol.* 2013;51:R51–R64.

9. Barnard ND, Scialli AR, Turner-McGrievy G, Lanou AJ, Glass J. The effects of a low-fat, plant-based dietary intervention on body weight, metabolism, and insulin sensitivity. *Am J Med.* 2005;118:991–97.

10. Mishra S, Xu J, Agarwal U, Gonzales J, Levin S, Barnard ND. A multicenter randomized controlled trial of a plant-based nutrition program to reduce body weight and cardiovascular risk in the corporate setting: the GEICO study. *Eur J Clin Nutr.* 2013;67:718–24.

11. Hooper L, Abdelhamid A, Moore HJ, Douthwaite W, Skeaff CM, Summerbell CD. Effect of reducing total fat intake on body weight: systematic review and meta-analysis of randomised controlled trials and cohort studies. *BMJ.* 2012 Dec 6;345:e7666. doi: 10.1136/bmj.e7666.

12. Hooper L, Abdelhamid A, Bunn D, Brown T, Summerbell CD, Skeaff CM. Effects of total fat intake on body weight. *Cochrane Database Syst Rev.* 2015 Aug 7;8:CD011834. doi: 10.1002/14651858.CD011834.

13. Hall KD, Bemis T, Brychta R, et al. Calorie for calorie, dietary fat restriction results in more body fat loss than carbohydrate restriction in people with obesity. *Cell Metabolism.* 2015;22:427–36.

Chapter 3. How Cheese Keeps You Hooked

1. Schulte EM, Avena NM, Gearhardt AN. Which foods may be addictive? The roles of processing, fat content, and glycemic load. *PLoS One.* 2015;10(2):e0117959.

2. Spetter MS, Smeets PAM, de Graaf C, Viergever MA. Representation of sweet and salty taste intensity in the brain. *Chem Senses.* 2010;35:831–40.

3. Liedtke WB, McKinley MJ, Walker LL, et al. Relation of addiction genes to hypothalamic gene changes subserving genesis and gratification of a classic instinct, sodium appetite. *Proc Natl Acad Sci.* 2011;108:12509–14.

4. Agriculture Research Service, U.S. Department of Agriculture. National Nutrient Database for Standard Reference Release 28. Internet: Accessed April 29, 2016.

5. Bolt D. Independent Chief Inspector of Borders and Immigration. An inspection of border force operations at Manchester Airport. July–October 2015. April 2016. Internet: http://icinspector.independent.gov.uk/wp-content /uploads/2016/04/An-Inspection-of-Border-Force-Operations-at-Manchester -Airport-July–October-2015.pdf. Accessed April 16, 2016.

6. Jakobsson I, Lindberg T. Cow's milk proteins cause infantile colic in breast-fed infants: a double-blind crossover study. *Pediatrics.* 1983;71:268–71.

7. Clyne PS, Kulczycki A Jr. Human breast milk contains bovine IgG. Relationship to infant colic? *Pediatrics.* 1991;87:439–44.

8. Jarmołowska B, Teodorowicz M, Fiedorowicz E, Sienkiewicz-Szłapka E, Matysiewicz M, Kostyra E. Glucose and calcium ions may modulate the efficiency of bovine β-casomorphin-7 permeability through a monolayer of Caco-2 cells. *Peptides.* 2013;49:59–67.

9. Kost NV, Sokolov OY, Kurasova OB, Dmitriev AD, Tarakanova JN, Gab-aeva MV, et al. Beta-casomorphins-7 in infants on different types of feeding and different levels of psychomotor development. *Peptides.* 2009;30(10):1854–60.

10. European Food Safety Authority. Review of the potential health impact of β-casomorphins and related peptides. Report of the DATEX Working Group on β-casomorphins. EFSA Scientific Report. 2009;231:1–107.

11. Lindström LH, Nyberg F, Terenius L, et al. CSF and plasma β-casomorphin-like opioid peptides in postpartum psychosis. *Am J Psychiatry.* 1984;141(9):1059–66.

12. Nyberg F, Lieberman H, Lindström LH, Lyrenäs S, Koch G, Terenius L. Immunoreactive β-casomorphin-8 in cerebrospinal fluid from pregnant and lactating women: correlation with plasma levels. *J Clin Endocr Metab.* 1989;68:283–89.

13. American Psychiatric Association. (2013). *Diagnostic and Statistical Manual of Mental Disorders* (5th ed.). Washington, DC.

14. Hetherington MM, MacDiarmid JI. "Chocolate addiction": a preliminary study of its description and its relationship to problem eating. *Appetite.* 1993 Dec;21(3):233–46.

Chapter 4. Hidden Hormone Effects

1. Manson JE, Chlebowski RT, Stefanick ML, et al. Menopausal hormone therapy and health outcomes during the intervention and extended post-stopping phases of the Women's Health Initiative randomized trials. *JAMA.* 2013;310(13):1353–68.

2. Premarin home page. Internet: https://www.premarin.com. Accessed November 30, 2015.

3. Pape-Zambito DA, Magliaro AL, Kensinger RS. Beta-estradiol and estrone concentrations in plasma and milk during bovine pregnancy. *J Dairy Sci.* 2008 Jan;91(1):127–35; Macrina AL, Ott TL, Roberts RF, Kensinger RS. Estrone and estrone sulfate concentrations in milk and milk fractions. *J Acad Nutr Diet.* 2012; 112(7):1088–93.

4. Hansen M, Halloran JM, Groth E, Lefferts LY. Potential public health impacts of the use of recombinant bovine somatotropin in dairy production. Consumers Union, September 1997. Internet: http://consumersunion .org/news/potential-public-health-impacts-of-the-use-of-recombinant-bovine -somatotropin-in-dairy-production-part-1/. Accessed March 29, 2016.

5. Brinkman MT, Baglietto L, Krishnan K, et al. Consumption of animal products, their nutrient components and postmenopausal circulating steroid hormone concentrations. *Eur J Clin Nutr.* 2010;64(2):176–83.

6. Kroenke CH, Kwan ML, Sweeney C, Castillo A, Caan BJ. High- and low-fat dairy intake, recurrence, and mortality after breast cancer diagnosis. *J Natl Cancer Inst.* 2013;105:616–23.

7. Afeiche M, Williams PL, Mendiola J, Gaskins AJ, Jørgensen N, Swan SH, Chavarro JE. Dairy food intake in relation to semen quality and reproductive hormone levels among physically active young men. *Human Reproduction.* 2013;28(8):2265–75.

8. Afeiche MC, Bridges ND, Williams PL, et al. Dairy intake and semen quality among men attending a fertility clinic. *Fertil Steril.* 2014;101(5):1280–87.

9. Barnard ND, Scialli AR, Hurlock D, Bertron P. Diet and sex-hormone binding globulin, dysmenorrhea, and premenstrual symptoms. *Obstet Gynecol.* 2000 Feb;95:245–50.

10. Wu AH, Yu MC, Tseng CC, Pike MC. Epidemiology of soy exposures and breast cancer risk. *Br J Cancer.* 2008;98:9–14.

11. Chen M, Rao Y, Zheng Y, et al. Association between soy isoflavone intake and breast cancer risk for pre- and post-menopausal women: a meta-analysis of epidemiological studies. *PLoS One.* 2014;9(2):e89288.

12. Nechuta SJ, Caan BJ, Chen WY, et al. Soy food intake after diagnosis of breast cancer and survival: an in-depth analysis of combined evidence from cohort studies of US and Chinese women. *Am J Clin Nutr.* 2012;96:123–32.

13. Ganmaa D, Li X, Wang J, Qin L, Wang P, Sato A. Incidence and mortality of testicular and prostatic cancers in relation to world dietary practices. *Int J Cancer.* 2002;98:262–67.

14. Chan JM, Stampfer MJ, Ma J, Gann PH, Gaziano JM, Giovannucci EL. Dairy products, calcium, and prostate cancer risk in the Physicians' Health Study. *Am J Clin Nutr.* 2001;74:549–54.

15. Giovannucci E, Rimm EB, Wolk A, et al. Calcium and fructose intake in relation to risk of prostate cancer. *Cancer Res.* 1998;58:442–47.

16. Heaney RP, McCarron DA, Dawson-Hughes B, et al. Dietary changes favorably affect bone remodeling in older adults. *J Am Dietetic Asso.* 1999; 99:1228–33.

17. Chan JM, Stampfer MJ, Giovannucci E, et al. Plasma insulin-like growth factor-I and prostate cancer risk: a prospective study. *Science.* 1998; 279:563–66.

18. Ornish D, Weidner G, Fair WR, et al. Intensive lifestyle changes may affect the progression of prostate cancer. *J Urol.* 2005;174:1065–69.

Chapter 5. Health Problems You Never Bargained For

1. National Asthma Council Australia. Dairy Products. Internet: http://www.nationalasthma.org.au/publication/dairy-products. Accessed February 22, 2016.

2. Thiara G, Goldman RD. Milk consumption and mucus production in children with asthma. *Can Fam Phys.* 2012;58:165–66.

3. Haas F, Bishop MC, Salazar-Schicchi J, Axen KV, Lieberman D, Axen K. Effect of milk ingestion on pulmonary function in healthy and asthmatic subjects. *J Asthma.* 1991;28(5):349–55.

4. Yusoff NA, Hampton SM, Dickerson JW, Morgan JB. The effects of exclusion of dietary egg and milk in the management of asthmatic children: a pilot study. *J R Soc Promot Health.* 2004;124(2):74–80.

5. Woods RK, Weiner JM, Abramson M, Thien F, Walters EH. Do dairy products induce bronchoconstriction in adults with asthma? *J Allergy Clin Immunol.* 1998;101(1 Pt 1):45–50; Nguyen MT. Effect of cow milk on pulmonary function in atopic asthmatic patients. *Ann Allergy Asthma Immunol.* 1997;79(1):62–64.

6. Greene HL, Hazlett D, Demaree R. Relation between Intralipid-induced hyperlipemia and pulmonary function. *Am J Clin Nutr.* 1976;29:127–35; Sundström G, Zauner CW, Aborelius M Jr: Decrease in pulmonary diffusing capacity during lipid infusion in healthy men. *J Appl Physiol.* 1973;34:816–20.

7. Haas F, Bishop MC, Salazar-Schicchi J, Axen KV, Lieberman D, Axen K. Effect of milk ingestion on pulmonary function in healthy and asthmatic subjects. *J Asthma.* 1991;28(5):349–55.

8. Bernstein JM. The role of IgE-mediated hypersensitivity in the development of otitis media with effusion. *Otolaryngol Clin North Am.* 1992;25(1): 197–211; James JM. Common respiratory manifestations of food allergy: a critical focus on otitis media. *Curr Allergy Asthma Rep.* 2004;4(4):294–301.

9. Egger J, Carter CM, Wilson J, Turner MW, Soothill JF. Is migraine food allergy? A double-blind controlled trial of oligoantigenic diet treatment. *Lancet*. 1983; 2:865–69.

10. Mansfield LE, Vaughan TR, Waller SF, Haverly RW, Ting S. Food allergy and adult migraine: double-blind and mediator confirmation of an allergic etiology. *Ann Allergy.* 1983;55:126–29.

11. Bic Z, Blix GG, Hopp HP, Leslie FM, Schell MJ. The influence of a low-fat diet on incidence and severity of migraine headaches. *J Womens Health Gend Based Med*. 1999;8:623–30.

12. Barnard ND, Scialli AR, Hurlock D, Bertron P. Diet and sex-hormone binding globulin, dysmenorrhea, and premenstrual symptoms. *Obstet Gynecol.* 2000 Feb;95(2):245–50.

13. Bunner AE, Agarwal U, Gonzales JF, Valente F, Barnard ND. Nutrition intervention for migraine: a randomized crossover trial. *J Headache Pain*. 2014 Oct 23;15:69.

14. Chandran V, Raychaudhuri SP. Geoepidemiology and environmental factors of psoriasis and psoriatic arthritis. *J Autoimmun*. 2010;34(3): J314–21.

15. Chandran V, Raychaudhuri SP. Geoepidemiology and environmental factors of psoriasis and psoriatic arthritis. *J Autoimmun*. 2010;34(3): J314–21.

16. Kjeldsen-Kragh J, Haugen M, Borchgrevink CF, et al. Controlled trial of fasting and one-year vegetarian diet in rheumatoid arthritis. *Lancet.* 1991;338(8772):899–902.

17. Hafström I, Ringertz B, Spångberg A, et al. A vegan diet free of gluten improves the signs and symptoms of rheumatoid arthritis: the effects on arthritis correlate with a reduction in antibodies to food antigens. *Rheumatology (Oxford)*. 2001;40(10):1175–79.

18. McDougall J, Bruce B, Spiller G, Westerdahl J, McDougall M. Effects of a very low-fat, vegan diet in subjects with rheumatoid arthritis. *J Altern Complement Med*. 2002;8(1):71–75.

19. Tilley BJ, Cook JL, Docking SI, Gaida JE. Is higher serum cholesterol associated with altered tendon structure or tendon pain? A systematic review. *Br J Sports Med*. 2015;49(23):1504–9.

20. Rob Demovsky. Aaron Rodgers cuts dairy products out of diet, now down to '218-ish'. ESPN. Internet: http://espn.go.com/nfl/story/_/id/16002518/aaron-rodgers-green-bay-packers-cuts-dairy-diet. Accessed June 9, 2016.

21. Cordain L, Lindeberg S, Hurtado M, Hill K, Eaton SB, Brand-Miller J. Acne vulgaris: a disease of Western civilization. *Archives of Dermatology*. 2002;138(12):1584–90.

22. Adebamowo CA, Spiegelman D, Danby FW, Frazier AL, Willett WC, Holmes MD. High school dietary intake and teenage acne. *J Am Acad Dermatol.* 2005;52:207–14.

23. Adebamowo CA, Spiegelman D, Berkey CS, et al. Milk consumption and acne in adolescent girls. *Dermatol Online J.* 2006;12(4):1–13; Adebamowo CA, Spiegelman D, Berkey CS, et al. Milk consumption and acne in teenaged boys. *J Am Acad Dermatol.* 2008;58(5):787–93.

24. Iacono G, Cavataio F, Montalto G, et al. Intolerance of cow's milk and chronic constipation in children. *N Engl J Med.* 1998;339:1100–4.

25. Karjalainen J, Martin JM, Knip M, et al. A bovine albumin peptide as a possible trigger of insulin-dependent diabetes mellitus. *N Engl J Med.* 1992;327:302–7.

26. Akerblom HK, Virtanen SM, Ilonen J, et al. Dietary manipulation of beta cell autoimmunity in infants at increased risk of type 1 diabetes: a pilot study. *Diabetologia.* 2005;48:829–37.

Chapter 6. Heart Disease, Diabetes, and the French Paradox

1. Roden M, Price TB, Perseghin G, Falk-Petersen K, Cline GW, Rothman DL, Shulman GI. Mechanism of free fatty acid-induced insulin resistance in humans. *J Clin Invest.* 1996;97:2859–65.

2. Hirabara SM, Curi R, Maechler P. Saturated fatty acid-induced insulin resistance is associated with mitochondrial dysfunction in skeletal muscle cells. *J Cell Physiol.* 2010;222:187–94.

3. Ornish D, Brown SE, Scherwitz LW, Billings JH, Armstrong WT, Ports TA, et al. Can lifestyle changes reverse coronary heart disease? *Lancet.* 1990;336:129–33.

4. Ornish D, Scherwitz LW, Billings JH, Brown SE, Gould KL, Merritt TA, Sparler S, Armstrong WT, Ports TA, Kirkeeide RL, Hogeboom C, Brand RJ. Intensive lifestyle changes for reversal of coronary heart disease. *JAMA.* 1998;280:2001–7; Yokoyama Y, Nishimura K, Barnard ND, Takegami M, Watanabe M, Sekikawa A, Okamura T, Miyamoto Y. Vegetarian diets and blood pressure: a meta-analysis. *JAMA Internal Medicine.* 2014;174(4):577–87; Barnard ND, Levin SM, Yokoyama Y. A systematic review and meta-analysis of changes in body weight in clinical trials of vegetarian diets. *J Acad Nutr Diet.* 2015 Jun;115(6):954–69.

5. U.S. Department of Agriculture National Agricultural Library. Internet: http://ndb.nal.usda.gov/ndb/foods/list.

6. U.S. Department of Agriculture Agricultural Research Service. USDA Food Composition Databases. Internet: http://ndb.nal.usda.gov/ndb/foods /list. Accessed September 12, 2016.

7. Morris MC, Evans EA, Bienias JL, et al. Dietary fats and the risk of incident Alzheimer's disease. *Arch Neurol.* 2003;60:194–200.

8. Eskelinen MH. Fat intake at midlife and cognitve impairment later in life: a population-based study. *Int J Geriatric Psychiatr.* 2008;23:741–47.

9. Solomon A, Kivipelto M, Wolozin B, Zhou J, Whitmer RA. Midlife serum cholesterol and increased risk of Alzheimer's and vascular dementia three decades later. *Dement Geriatr Cogn Disord.* 2009;28:75–80.

10. Law M, Wald N. Why heart disease mortality is low in France: the time lag explanation. *BMJ.* 1999;318:1471–76.

11. Law M, Wald N. Why heart disease mortality is low in France: the time lag explanation. *BMJ.* 1999;318:1471–76.

12. Law M, Wald N. Why heart disease mortality is low in France: the time lag explanation. *BMJ.* 1999;318:1471–76.

13. Law M, Wald N. Why heart disease mortality is low in France: the time lag explanation. *BMJ.* 1999;318:1471–76.

14. Cuisine française les principales différences entre les régions, help ! Aufeminin. Internet: http://forum.aufeminin.com/forum/cuisine1/__f119892 _cuisine1-Cuisine-francaise-les-principales-differences-entre-les-regions-help .html. Accessed June 9, 2016.

15. Law M, Wald N. Why heart disease mortality is low in France: the time lag explanation. *BMJ.* 1999;318:1471–76.

16. Vicky Buffery. Real French women really do get fat. Reuters. November 10, 2009. Internet: http://www.reuters.com/article/lifestyleMolt/idUSTRE5A 93I220091110. Accessed June 9, 2016.

17. Fodor GJ, Helis E, Yazdekhasti N, Vohnout B. "Fishing" for the origins of the "Eskimos and heart disease" story: facts or wishful thinking? A review. *Can J Cardiol.* 2014;30(8):864–68.

18. Mann GV. The Masai, milk and the yogurt factor: an alternative explanation. *Atherosclerosis.* 1978;29:265.

19. Keys A. Atherosclerosis: a problem in newer public health. *J Mt Sinai Hosp NY.* 1953;20:118–39.

20. Ycrushalmy J, Hilleboe HE. Fat in the diet and mortality from heart disease: a methodologic note. *NY State J Med.* 1957;57:2343–54.

21. Chowdhury R, Warnakula S, Kunutsor S, et al. Association of dietary, circulating, and supplement fatty acids with coronary risk: a systematic review and meta-analysis. *Ann Intern Med.* 2014;160:398–406.

22. Appleby PN, Thorogood M, Mann JI, Key TJA. The Oxford Vegetarian Study: an overview. *Am J Clin Nutr.* 1999;70(suppl):525S–531S.

23. Wallström P, Sonestedt E, Hlebowicz J, Ericson U, Drake I, Persson M, et al. Dietary fiber and saturated fat intake associations with cardiovascular disease differ by sex in the Malmö Diet and Cancer Cohort: a prospective study. *PLoS One.* 2012;7:e31637.

24. Editorial board. Scientists get egg on their faces. *Chicago Tribune.* Internet: http://www.chicagotribune.com/news/opinion/editorials/ct-cholesterol -guidelines-edit-0223-20150220-story.html. Accessed November 9, 2016.

25. Mark Bittman. How should we eat? *New York Times.* Internet: http://www.nytimes.com/2015/02/25/opinion/how-should-we-eat.html. Accessed June 17, 2016.

26. Food and Nutrition Board, Institute of Medicine. Dietary Reference Intakes for Energy, Carbohydrate, Fiber, Fat, Fatty Acids, Cholesterol, Protein, and Amino Acids. Washington, DC: National Academies Press; 2002/2005.

Chapter 7. What the Animals Go Through

1. Food and Agriculture Organization of the United Nations. *Small-Scale Dairy Farming Manual,* 2008. Internet: http://www.fao.org/docrep/011/t1265e /t1265e.htm. Accessed April 30, 2016. Reproduced with permission.

2. Dave Rogers. Strange noises turn out to be cows missing their calves. *Daily News.* Newburyport, Mass. Internet: http://www.newburyportnews.com/ news/local_news/strange-noises-turn-out-to-be-cows-missing-their-calves/ article_d872e4da-b318-5e90-870e-51266f8eea7f.html. Accessed March 27, 2016.

3. Belanger Jerome D. and Sara Thomson Bredesen. *Storey's Guide to Raising Dairy Goats,* 4th edition. Storey Publishing, North Adams, MA, 2000, 2001.

Chapter 8. The Industry Behind the Addiction

1. Dairy Management Inc. Dairy Checkoff leader tells farmers from across the country how they can help grow sales and trust. November 14, 2013. Internet: http://www.dairy.org/news/2013/november/dairy-checkoff-leader -tells-farmers-from-across-the-country-how-they-can-help-grow-sales-and -trust. Accessed March 12, 2016.

2. Zemel MB, Thompson W, Milstead A, Morris K, Campbell P. Calcium and dairy acceleration of weight and fat loss during energy restriction in obese adults. *Obes Res.* 2004;12(4):582–90.

3. Zemel MB, Richards J, Mathis S, Milstead A, Gebhardt L, Silva E. Dairy augmentation of total and central fat loss in obese subjects. *Int J Obes (Lond).* 2005;29(4):391–97.

4. Barr SI. Increased dairy product or calcium intake: is body weight or composition affected in humans? *J Nutr*. 2003;133:245S–48S.

5. Lanou AJ, Barnard ND. Dairy and weight loss hypothesis: an evaluation of the clinical trials. *Nutr Rev*. 2008;66(5):272–79.

6. Lloyd T, Petit MA, Lin HM, Beck TJ. Lifestyle factors and the development of bone mass and bone strength in young women. *J Pediatr*. 2004; 144(6):776–82.

7. Lanou AJ, Berkow S, Barnard ND. Calcium, dairy products, and bone health in children and young adults: a reevaluation of the evidence. *Pediatrics*. 2005;115:736–43.

8. Feskanich D, Willett WC, Colditz GA. Calcium, vitamin D, milk consumption, and hip fractures: a prospective study among postmenopausal women. *Am J Clin Nutr*. 2003;77(2):504–11.

9. Feskanich D, Bischoff-Ferrari HA, Frazier AL, Willett WC. Milk consumption during teenage years and risk of hip fractures in older adults. *JAMA Pediatr*. 2014;168(1):54–60.

10. Maryland Technology Enterprise Institute. Concussion-related measures improved in high school football players who drank new chocolate milk, UMD study shows. Internet: http://www.mtech.umd.edu/news/press _releases/releases/5QF/concussions/. Accessed March 19, 2016.

11. University of Maryland School of Public Health, Department of Kinesiology. Jae Kun Shim. Internet: https://sph.umd.edu/department/knes/faculty/people /jae-kun-shim. Accessed: November 8, 2016.

12. Academy of Nutrition and Dietetics website. Meet Our Sponsors. Internet: http://www.eatrightpro.org/resources/about-us/advertising-and-sponsorship /meet-our-sponsors. Accessed June 3, 2016.

13. Academy of Nutrition and Dietetics/Foundation. Fiscal Year 2015 Annual Report. Internet: http://www.eatrightpro.org/~/media/eatrightpro%20files/ about%20us/annual%20reports/annualreport2015.ashx. Accessed June 3, 2016.

14. American Academy of Pediatrics. Friends of Children Fund Corporate Member News. Internet: https://www.aap.org/en-us/about-the-aap/corporate -relationships/Pages/Friends-of-Children-Fund-Corporate-Member-News .aspx. Accessed June 9, 2016.

15. USDA Report to Congress on the National Dairy Promotion and Research Program and the National Fluid Milk Processor Promotion Program. July 1, 2006. Internet: https://www.ams.usda.gov/sites/default/files/media/2005%20 -%20Dairy%20Report%20to%20Congress.pdf. Accessed March 20, 2015.

16. Dietitians for Professional Integrity. Internet: http://integritydietitians .org. Accessed May 3, 2016.

Index

About the Author

Neal D. Barnard, MD, FACC, is an adjunct associate professor of medicine at the George Washington University School of Medicine in Washington, DC, and president of the Physicians Committee for Responsible Medicine.

Dr. Barnard has led numerous research studies investigating the effects of diet on diabetes, body weight, and chronic pain, including a groundbreaking study of dietary interventions in type 2 diabetes, funded by the National Institutes of Health. Dr. Barnard has authored more than seventy scientific publications as well as eighteen books.

As president of the Physicians Committee for Responsible Medicine, Dr. Barnard leads programs advocating for preventive medicine, good nutrition, and higher ethical standards in research. He has hosted three PBS television programs on nutrition and health and is frequently called on by news programs to discuss issues related to nutrition and research. He is the editor in chief of the *Nutrition Guide for Clinicians*, a textbook made available to all U.S. medical students. His research contributed to the acceptance of plant-based diets in the Dietary Guidelines for Americans. In 2015, he was named a Fellow of the American College of Cardiology.

Originally from Fargo, North Dakota, Dr. Barnard received his MD degree at the George Washington University School of Medicine and completed his residency at the same institution. He practiced at St. Vincent's Hospital in New York before returning to Washington to found the Physicians Committee.